"I've learned it's not the price of the ingredients or complexity of the process that is responsible for the success of the final product. Rather, it's technical skill melded with precision and patience that makes the difference between a disaster and a delicacy."
—From *Cheapskate in the Kitchen*

Mary Hunt learned it the hard way. After years of paying for Chinese takeout, frozen dinners, and restaurant fare, she made the leap from being a slave to overpriced "convenience" foods to mistress of her domain—a gourmet kitchen in her own home—creating superb meals for her family on a shoestring budget.

You can, too, with *Cheapskate Gourmet*. It's the only guide you'll need to stock a basic, functional kitchen; experiment with and practice new skills; learn to cut food costs while not skimping on taste and satisfaction; and share the many benefits—including the financial rewards—with your entire family.

Get ready to save—and to dine better than ever—with *Cheapskate Gourmet*.

Mary Hunt's
CHEAPSKATE
G·O·U·R·M·E·T

Mary Hunt's
CHEAPSKATE
G·O·U·R·M·E·T

Creating Fabulous Meals
for a Fraction of the Cost

BROADMAN
&HOLMAN
PUBLISHERS

Nashville, Tennessee

0-8054-2443-1

Published by Broadman & Holman Publishers, Nashville, Tennessee

Dewey Decimal Classification: 641.5
Subject Heading: COOKING / ENTERTAINING
Library of Congress Card Catalog Number: 00-067471

Library of Congress Cataloging-in-Publication Data
Hunt, Mary, 1948–
    [Cheap-skate in the Kitchen]
    Mary Hunt's cheapskate gourmet : creating fabulous meals
for a fraction of the cost / Mary Hunt.
        p. cm.
    Previously published as: Cheap-skate in the kitchen. 1997.
    Includes bibliographical references and index.
    ISBN 0-8054-2443-1 (pb.)
    1. Low budget cookery. I. Title.
TX652.H859   2001
641.5'52—dc21

                                            00-067471

                                                CIP

3 4 5 6 7 8 9 10 05 04 03 02 01

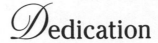Dedication

*This book is lovingly dedicated to the two people
in my life who most perfectly embody a true gourmet.*

To my grandmother, *Mamie Schwartz,* who always prepared meals that were as lovely as she was. Never did a person enter her home who was not offered delectable food—a clear affirmation of that person's value. Grandma, you modeled for me the attributes of a truly beautiful woman, and I miss you more than words can tell.

To my sister-in-law, *Marilyn McCormick,* who more than anyone I have ever known can turn plain, boring food into unbelievable works of art. I recall with clarity each meal I've eaten at your table, the tastes of which will remain in my memory forever. Marilyn, through your example you have taught me how to value the simple and elevate the ordinary.

$\mathcal{C}$ontents

Acknowledgments

Many people have contributed greatly in making this book possible. Cathy Hollenbeck researched, collaborated, and assisted from the first moment to the release of the manuscript. Barbara Nosek, Bob Kingsbury, Judy Bergman, Marilyn McCormick, Mary Ann Woirhaye, Patrick Schroeder, Paulette Hegg, Jan Sandberg, Ray and Nancy Guth, Margaret F. Gamble, Debi Taylor-Hough, Eunice Douglas, Dorothy Carnine, Julia Wright, Betty Coates, June Rich, and Alice Cook responded to many questions and were kind enough to share their thoughts, secrets, and recipes. Karen Wayman, Sue Hoby, Chris Williams, Mary Evers, Teri Pickering, Barbara Bectel, Liz Blough, Julie Harper, and Marilyn Trimmer contributed favorite gourmet recipes.

A million thanks to each one of you. Please take great pride in this book because your involvement was very important in the entire process.

Special thanks to my husband, Harold, for thinking anything I cook is a masterpiece; my son, Josh, for sharing my love of cole slaw and California Roll, and my son; Jeremy, for keeping me in stitches even when it appears I'm not at all amused.

My Collaborator

Before you turn another page, you must meet my collaborator, Cathy Hollenbeck. I first met Cathy when I interviewed her for an administrative position in the real estate company my husband and I own. It didn't take long for us to recognize this woman was born to manage our busy office. Clearly she was overqualified but, even so, agreed to take the position.

Jump ahead to 1991. Real estate was on the decline in California; I was in need of a new passion—something fresh and exciting. In one of my many dreaming sessions, I selected something completely off-the-wall: to write and publish a monthly newsletter that I would title *Cheapskate Monthly*. Fortunately, my plans were developing so quickly I failed to consider I knew nothing about either aspect, publishing or writing. Had I pondered that fact, I might not have proceeded due to sheer terror.

It was a day I shall not soon forget. I walked into the office and announced to Cathy that we were going to publish a newsletter. Used to my eccentricities, she politely humored me. She remained loyal and cautiously enthusiastic about our new endeavor and as encouraging as she could be in light of such a wacky change of direction. However, when the media started calling, checks began to roll in, our mailbox overflowed day after day, and the subscriber list started growing like a weed in hot sunshine, Cathy threw caution to the wind and wholeheartedly joined me for the ride of a lifetime.

Little did I care when I first hired her that she held degrees in journalism and marketing from the prestigious University of Southern California. Suddenly I cared a lot and concluded that, in truth, she was born to be my senior editor, assistant, media liaison, and all-around editorial manager. That was justification enough for me to steal her from the real estate office.

I've learned many things about Cathy over the years, not the least of which is this: She is a fabulous gourmet cook. When the idea of this book came to me, I jumped into the nebulous possibility with all-fours only to panic when my editor, Jennifer Weis, at St. Martin's Press, accepted my proposal. In a single moment I got my green light to proceed and a deadline to meet.

Once again Cathy came to my rescue and jumped right in. She contributed so much from her own wealth of knowledge and experience and coordinated all communications between me and the many gourmet cooks you are going to meet in the pages that follow.

Cathy, I could have never completed this book without you. You are a loyal employee, a passionate publicist, and best of all, my very dear friend. Thank you from the bottom of my heart.

$\mathcal{I}$ntroduction

Hi there, and welcome to my book. What kind of book is this? you ask. Well, it is not a newfangled plan for getting dinner on the table in ten minutes, start to finish. And it's not a gourmet *cookbook*. This is a book that will teach you how to get from Spaghetti-Os to Scallopini alla Marsala, culinarily speaking. It's for those who don't have the knowledge to be Cordon Bleu chefs, let alone the money to purchase expensive ingredients and equipment. It's for those who have noticed the tremendous growth in the interest of food and cooking—evidenced by the increase of specialty stores, gourmet sections of grocery stores, food magazines, cookbooks, cooking classes, and professional chef training schools—and long to participate but don't know how to "get with the program."

This is a book for those who yearn to prepare and present meals with all the style of Martha Stewart, the talent of Julia Child, the delightful wit of Graham Kerr, and the expertise of Christopher Kimball. It's for those who go on day after day, secretly wishing and yearning to be fine gourmet cooks, but find themselves stuck in the macaroni-and-cheese rut, hanging onto a dream that someday, somehow, they'll magically make that quantum leap from wieners to Wolfgang.

Well, my friend, that day has arrived. And the best news of all is you won't need to get an extra job or win the lottery to be a gourmet. In fact, you're going to find that you actually spend less money whenever you ditch prepackaged, preprepared meals chock-full of preservatives and unpronounceable chemicals. The closer you can get to preparing meals using pure, natural, raw ingredients (also known as cooking from scratch) the more money you'll save and the more healthy meals you and your family will eat.

Now don't panic. Just because you may not be able to devote the time necessary each day to this new undertaking doesn't mean you can't get started. Just start out slowly. Maybe you can begin by creating one fabulous meal each weekend. Practice, practice, and practice some more until you are an expert at one particular technique, such as making the perfect pâté brisée (pie crust) or hollandaise (sauce). Then add another technique and another special recipe, and before you know it you'll be hooked. Your gourmet cooking will spill over into other days of the week. Friends and relatives will anxiously await your dinner invitations, and your family will feel abused those times they are forced to go out to eat. OK, that might be stretching it a bit, but you get my point.

I'm so glad you picked up this book, and I know you won't be disappointed. This is not a cookbook for those few who are already skilled in the art of gourmet cooking. It is a guide, an easy-to-read collection of the basics, the step-by-step how-tos and techniques plus lots of tricks from masters of the trade for those who desire to become gourmet cooks. We'll cover everything you need to know so that you don't bust the budget in the process of developing a new skill. I will explain in specific details exactly how to perform each technique.

If I, somewhat of a kitchen klutz myself, can perfect a world-class brioche, so can you. And even though this isn't exactly a cookbook, I will share a plethora of wonderful recipes to get you going.

So whether it's Martha's or Julia's, Graham's, Christopher's, or Wolfgang's—or even your mother's cooking—you wish to emulate, fasten your apron, rev up your whisk, and let's get going!

Part One

The Classic Essentials
of Gourmet Cooking

*Why settle for mediocrity when it takes
so little effort to achieve excellence?*

Chapter One

*F*ood for Thought

Attitudes about food have changed dramatically since the 1960s when home economics was a required course for female junior high students. Back then the term *fast food* had not yet been coined and the idea of a microwave oven in every home was too outrageous to be taken seriously.

Fast-forward some thirty years to the present, and sure enough, those miraculous ovens we feared would "nuke" the house and everyone in it have become standard equipment in the typical American kitchen. Fast-food joints have sprung up in every nook and cranny of our cities, and baby's first words are more likely to be *French fries* than *da-da* or *ma-ma*.

We live in an age when "instantly" is not quite soon enough. Overnight mail seems unacceptably slow now that we are used to two-second E-mail transmissions. We've become mesmerized by the allure of instant cash, instant credit, and instant gratification. As a whole, this nation has become hooked on convenience, and we are willing to go to some pretty amazing lengths to have it. No wonder we've been dubbed the microwave generation—a society of individuals who feel entitled to have everything right now, if not sooner.

I have been known to race into the house an hour late; program the microwave to defrost and heat preformed, fully cooked, hormone-injected chicken patties containing artificial chicken flavoring; tear open a uniquely breathable plastic bag of who-knows-how-old ready-to-eat salad greens; toss it together with an ample glob of nonfat, no-cholesterol, nondairy Ranchlike dressing (I think it's really Spackle with a hint of artificial sweetener); pop a loaf of pre-cut, garlic butter–flavored bread complete with artificial herblike seasonings (and a shelf life of five years) into a preheated cyclonic-action oven; and have dinner on the table in 7.2 minutes flat. Yum.

Ah, technology. Who knows where it will take us next? Trust me. I love this high-tech age and would not go back to the 1960s for anything. I'm fascinated by the latest in amazing electronic gadgets and scientific progress. I'll never figure out how a signal can be beamed into the sky halfway around the world so precisely that it hits a bull's-eye on a satellite (which is, by the way, the relative size of a speck of dust), bounce that signal back to earth without it getting hopelessly tangled with other signals, position it with such accuracy that it hits a tiny cable that runs into my home, and then convert it into a color picture that is straight and right-side-up not on the refrigerator but right on the television screen! And all in a matter of seconds. That's just too cool for words.

I wish that whoever is in charge of new technology would get into high gear on an affordable self-cleaning house. Just imagine leaving in the morning, tossing a few gallons of automatic house-washing detergent through the mail slot, selecting the heavy-duty cycle, throwing the lever into locked position, and driving away knowing that when you return your home and contents will be sparkling clean with no embarrassing water spots.

When I step back and look at the big picture, I see quite a dilemma and wonder if you've noticed it too. On the one hand we're privileged to live in the most progressive and exciting time this nation has ever known. I wouldn't suggest for a moment that we regress to living off the land, refusing to partake in modern conveniences. I, for one, am pretty hooked on electricity, automobiles, computers, and yes, even that invisible indescribable thing out there in space called the Internet.

But on the other hand our lives are so fast paced and our schedules so tightly packed, somedays we don't know if we're coming or going let alone if the entire family will ever again land in the same room at the same time. It's a wonder that with all our spinning out of control we don't propel ourselves right off the planet.

It occurs to me that the solution may be found in having a personal pressure valve that provides instant (of course) relief when life becomes hectic beyond reason. I'd like to suggest that capitalizing on one of the most delightful parts of civilized life—the pleasures of the table—is one way we can offer that kind of haven to ourselves, our families, and our friends.

The best refuge you could ever hope for is right there in the warmth and security of your home; where the basic human need for what is healthy, delicious, familiar, and comforting can be filled; where food is graciously presented.

The Spirituality of Food

When we offer someone food, we are not just giving that guest something to eat; we are giving far more. We give strength, health, beauty, clarity of mind, and even life because none of those things would be possible without food. So when we feed another, this is what we are offering—the substance of life itself.

In a single moment of offering food, our spirituality comes into play. Loving-kindness is there because we feel goodwill toward the person who is receiving, and we want him or her to be happy. We feel compassion in that moment because we wish our guest to be free from pain or suffering. We experience sympathetic joy, rejoicing in the person's happiness and wanting it to increase. Equanimity manifests in the act of giving because we are willing to let go of something we have; we are willing to be without it ourselves.

In that one instant of giving, we also abandon the tormentors of our hearts. We let go of desire and greed. We abandon ill will or aversion, a state that creates separateness, distance, withdrawal. And we abandon delusion, because when we perform a wholesome or skillful action like giving, we understand that what we do in our lives—

the choices we make, the values we hold—all count for something. Surely this must be the true essence of "it is in giving that we receive."

The connection between food and spirituality is as old as the Bible itself and yet timely as though torn from today's headlines. We "hunger and thirst after righteousness"; we "find the Lord a sweet savor"; we "taste and see that He is good"; we "desire the sincere milk of the word."

Surely, sharing food is a metaphor for all giving.

Food as an Art Form

Seeing food as an art form is one of the more delightful parts of civilized life. A well-prepared and presented meal has the ability to create feelings of calm, waves of joy, and a sense of well-being.

It's easy to argue that you don't have the time, resources, or ability to devote to culinary pleasure. The truth is, all of us make time for those things that are of a high priority. And resources? Preparing food from scratch is much less costly than buying it preprepared. And when it comes to food preparation, ability means a desire to learn the basics and then commit to perfecting the skill. Natural talent is not necessarily a prerequisite for becoming a gourmet cook.

A New Generation

If you are part of the current generation of heat-'n'-eat cooks who did not grow up in the classic traditions of food preparation, don't despair. It's not too late to learn what you've missed. If I can, I'm certain you can too.

The sum total of what I knew about food preparation the day I crossed the threshold into our first home—complete with my very own, albeit microscopic, kitchen—I learned from my home economics teacher, Mrs. Gilkey. Bless her heart, she did her best to teach us simple basics, and with great success I might add. I completed her foods class with a decent grade and adequate confidence to prepare three masterpieces: cinnamon toast, scrambled eggs, and pie crust.

My culinary repertoire developed only minimally until quite a few years later. About twenty to be exact.

During those interim years I graduated from college, married, and gave birth to two sons of average size and one king-sized amount of consumer debt (another story on its own). We'd hit bottom, financially speaking, and in my desperation to keep from losing the things that really mattered to me (things like my home and family), I was all but forced to start cooking—from *scratch*—in an attempt to slash our exorbitant monthly food bill. I had no way to anticipate the fringe benefits of such a noble endeavor.

I wasn't an overnight sensation in the kitchen (the truth is, I've still not reached sensational) and, for lack of a better plan of action, picked up right where Mrs. Gilkey left off. I used scrambled eggs as a springboard to conquer omelets. My cinnamon toast was a perfect lead-in to cinnamon rolls. Knowing how to make an excellent pâté brisée (pie crust to the common cook) presented all kinds of options from quiches to mile-high lemon curd pie. It wasn't difficult to add these dishes to my résumé.

The most difficult thing for me wasn't the chopping, braising, whipping, or sautéing. It was changing my attitude, which was far more challenging. I felt put upon, poor, and destitute for having to spend so much time in the kitchen. Inside, I was dying to order Chinese takeout or make my favorite thing for dinner (reservations).

In time I began to turn out honest-to-goodness homemade meals that were quite a treat for a family so sick of eating out. It felt good, and I was pretty proud of myself. I started simply and little by little picked up new techniques, which boosted my confidence. I was rewarded with lower food costs, increased personal satisfaction, and an unexplainable new fondness for my progress toward gourmet cooking.

Saturday Afternoon Delight

Over the years I've been uniquely privileged to sit under the personal tutelage of world-famous gourmet cooks the likes of Julia Child, Christopher Kimball, Martha Stewart, Martin Yan, and Jacques

Pépin. Every weekend I have standing appointments with one or more of them. They come right into my home and demonstrate unique techniques while I assume a prone position, curled up in my favorite blanket, first-row-center in front of the television.

They've taught me that it takes practice, practice, and more practice to become good at anything, especially serious cooking. They constantly give me permission to try, try, and try again. Chucking an occasional failed attempt down the disposal doesn't feel as though I'm banned from trying again. On occasion I've tossed the mess out and started over three or four times in the same session before I finally got it right. What a feeling of accomplishment when it finally worked.

What Is a Gourmet Cook?

Here's my very broad definition: *A gourmet cook is one who fills the gap somewhere between a basically good cook and a French-trained chef.* (Many dear friends of mine who I consider to be gourmet cooks graciously shared their thoughts on the matter of gourmet cooking. One of my questions was, what is your definition of *a gourmet cook* and *a gourmet meal?* Their responses follow at the end of this chapter.)

A good cook is one who has the skill to prepare excellent-tasting food.

A gourmet cook is one who has the skills to prepare and present excellent-tasting, nonstereotypical foods in such a way that a meal becomes an occasion.

A chef is a gourmet cook who combines natural talent, formal training, and creative skills on a professional level and is paid to do so.

A beginning gourmet cook follows a recipe with impeccable accuracy, while a seasoned gourmet often takes liberties with recipes and modifies according to personal taste.

A gourmet cook highly regards the recipe, the ingredients, the process, and the results. Need proof? Just listen to Graham or Julia— or read their classic tomes. They can rhapsodize for hours on the beauty of a perfect beet, the gleam on an eggplant. Over and over again you'll see one of them stroke a perfectly deboned, defatted, and deskinned chicken and fawn over a gloriously smooth and rich sauce. With all the sincerity in the world, these delightful souls often declare an ingredient or finished product to be "absolutely gorgeous." They cradle a copper bowl in the bend of an elbow, looking deep into its contents, amazed by its delicate beauty—much the same way a mother cradles and adores a newborn child.

Or how about Martha when she pronounces something she's just created to be a "good thing." These folks fall in love with a perfectly marbleized rump roast; they are filled with rapture upon finding produce so beautiful it must be dealt with immediately; they respect the qualities of yeast and gluten so deeply that they make sure the dough is allowed the perfectly proper amount of time to rest.

These fine gourmets have a keen sense of when to avoid or encourage chemical-type reactions when combining certain ingredients. Clearly, Jacques Pépin would never require a pastry to skip its chilling nap or for a hollandaise sauce to be heated quickly to hurry things along. My favorite gourmets just couldn't let themselves engage in activities quite so foolish.

I've learned the hard way how important it is to follow instructions. When a recipe instruction said to chill the dough for two hours, I'd skip that part. What's the point of chilling something that is bound for the oven anyway? Made no sense to me. And why dry off the chicken parts when they're just going to get wet again once they're dropped in oil or smothered with sauce?

When a recipe called for 1 cup plus 2 tablespoons flour, I'd do it my way to avoid getting another utensil dirty. What's the big deal about those extra 2 tablespoons of flour, anyway? I didn't feel that measurements needed to be so terribly accurate. Obviously, "plus 2 tablespoons" simply meant 1 cup of flour wasn't quite enough. Dumping in a little extra should have done the trick.

What I lacked in respect for the art of food preparation, I more than made up for in arrogance and a flippant attitude. But no matter what shortcut I chose or instruction I refused to follow, visions of Mrs. Gilkey and her insistence on impeccable technique always came to mind. I knew better, but for some reason I just didn't care. I was hardly on the road to being a gourmet—yet!

Why Become a Gourmet Cook?

Let me count the reasons:

Preparing and presenting glorious meals will give you a wonderful sense of well-being and acceptance. Face it, who among us doesn't enjoy a sincere compliment now and again? The approval of those we love and care about is very important for building and maintaining a sense of personal worth. Besides, it's kind of nice to own a special skill no one else in the family can duplicate.

Presenting a fine gourmet meal promotes good table manners and quality family time without verbal instruction or admonishment. It has a way of sending a silent instruction to kids to avail themselves of their best manners. I'd never considered this particular benefit until I happened to notice it in my own kids. Chowing down a lukewarm cheeseburger and soggy fries in front of the television for some reason doesn't command the respect and graciousness that is given to a succulently prepared, beautifully presented meal. When children observe adults partake of fine food around a dining table where the focus is the meal, not the evening news, they are more likely to become well-mannered, confident adults.

Presenting quality meals of a gourmet caliber delivers a very clear message about how much you care. It doesn't matter if you're entertaining the President or your precious teenager; the message comes across loud and clear without speaking a word.

Having the reputation of being a gourmet cook with a beautiful meal always at the ready can act as a magnet to fill "empty nests." If you want your grown children and friends to return home often and of their own accord, become a gourmet cook.

Where to Start?

I can't think of a better place than finishing this book. If you follow through by practicing techniques and actual step-by-step preparations, you'll have the jump-start you need to achieve the status of a gourmet cook. Gradually you'll build up your knowledge and confidence. Your store of learned techniques will increase, and soon you'll feel that you really are on your way to becoming a gourmet cook. In time the cookbook section of your library or bookstore will take on new meaning. You'll be eager to test new recipes and add equipment to your kitchen.

Start simply and don't create for yourself unrealistic expectations, even when you've completed this book and mastered many of the techniques and recipes. In other words, it's probably not a good idea to invite eight for dinner tomorrow night because you've been dying to tackle coulibiac of bass. Trust me, panic will set in like you've never experienced when you notice this particular culinary feast (which you won't find in this book but on page 224 of *The Martha Stewart Cookbook*) is very complicated and requires two days for preparation.

Start small. Prepare something wonderful just for yourself and maybe your family, first. Then build from there. Remember, a main ingredient in becoming a successful gourmet cook is confidence—confidence in the food, the presentation, and the consumption.

Indulgences

A new phobia has arisen over the past decade or two. Julia Child calls it *fear of food* and blames it on media hype and woefully inadequate information. Formulas for keeping fit and healthy change, not unlike current fashions and style. No matter what the current fad or trend, it seems we always come back to the idea of moderation in everything from pâtés to pickles, vitamins to fibrous cure-alls, butter lettuce to butter creams. Overdosing on anything brings trouble.

Some of the recipes found throughout this book include salt, butter, eggs, cheese, and cream. However, the focus is on moderation and balance rather than elimination. Today's great chefs have not eliminated these items from their repertoires but have instead reduced their dependence on them, turning much of their focus to herbs, spices, and flavoring agents for added flavoring, color, and texture in their food. It is their example we wish to emulate.

Julia Child offers a very wise, healthful, and balanced philosophy regarding indulgence, moderation, and variety.

An imaginary shelf labeled Indulgences *is a good idea. It contains the best butter, jumbo-sized eggs, heavy cream, marbled steak, sausages and pâtés, hollandaise and butter sauces, French butter-cream fillings, gooey chocolate cakes, and all those lovely items that demand disciplined rationing. Thus, with these items high up and almost out of reach, we are ever conscious that they are not everyday foods. They are for special occasions, and when those occasions come, we can enjoy every mouthful.*

Servings indicated in recipes are for conventional amounts, but for all of us it's sensible, indeed, to make a habit of smaller helpings. I, for one, would much rather swoon over a few thin slices of prime beefsteak, or one small serving of chocolate mousse, or a sliver of foie gras than indulge to the full on such nonentities as fat-free gelatin puddings.[1]

Nutritional Information

Most of the recipes that appear in part 2 of this book include basic nutritional data. It will not take the careful reader long to notice that many of the recipes fall into the category of *indulgences,* upon which one's steady diet should not be based.

I have included many recipes that should be reserved for creating occasions and memorable events. If you allow yourself to be guided by moderation and variety plus exercise and weight-watching, there's no reason you cannot eat a great variety of ordinary and fabulous foods.

I hope you will adopt Julia's philosophy when approaching the recipes in this book and that you will plan for and welcome them as guiltless indulgences. Let nothing hinder you from luxuriating from time to time in the joy and beauty of a beautifully conceived meal.

---

1. Julia Child, *The Way to Cook* (New York: Alfred A. Knopf, 1989), xi.

Comments from Our Panel of Gourmet Cooks in Response to "What Is Your Definition of a Gourmet Cook?"

A gourmet cook is one who has aced the finals on the basics and has gone on to attain some mastery of the more complex procedures. The gourmet cook can successfully stir in some personalized touches in the form of a just-right overlay ingredient, an inspired combination, or some flair in presentation!

— Barbara Nosek, Nevada

A gourmet cook is someone who cares enough to be creative in their cooking, preparation, and presentation of a meal.

—Bob Kingsbury, California

A gourmet cook is someone who knows all about fancy French names and strange herbs (grown in their kitchens) and creates wonderful smells that waft from their homes.

—Judy Bergman, California

A gourmet cook is one who can make and present ordinary food that tastes and looks good. This person appreciates a good meal.

—Marilyn McCormick, California

When thinking about the term gourmet cook, *French (especially the Cordon Bleu School of the Culinary Arts) and $$$ may come to mind. But as I always tell my kids, "Look in the dictionary!" The word* gourmet *used as a noun means "commissioner of food and drink." I've commissioned food and drink for my family (husband, self, three children, a grandfather, granddaughter, live-in aunt, kids' friends, and a few neighbors). I've been a gourmet cook six nights a week for thirty-two years.*

—Mary Ann Woirhaye, California

A gourmet cook is one who enjoys cooking creatively and sharing the results.

—Patrick Schroeder, California

A gourmet cook is someone who has mastered the art of cooking. It involves instinct, passion, creativity, a practical sense of knowing the "how-to" and what makes a dish special. A gourmet

cook is willing to try something new and is not afraid to take a risk.
—Jan Sandberg, California

My definition of a gourmet cook is one with the ability to turn a meal into an event.
—Paulette Hegg, Washington

I have always thought of a gourmet cook as one whose food is made with love and served with flair.
—Julia Wright, California

Gourmet food to me is food the way God intended it—to arrive via farmers not chemists. Gourmet food is real food!
—Dorothy Carnine, Nebraska

My guests refer to me as a Southern Gourmet which I take as a compliment. Gourmet to me means high quality, tasty food presented in a way to tantalize the taste buds before the first bite is ever taken.
—Margaret F. Gamble, Alabama
Author of *Tasty Creations Cookbook*

Here's my definition of gourmet: creativity in cooking, preparing, and serving a meal; not being confined to a recipe, but brave enough to alter it or invent a new one; usually starting from scratch; using the freshest of ingredients; cooking only to crisp-tender, al dente stage, so that vegetables retain their bright color, meats their moisture, and pastas their shape and texture.
—Eunice Douglas, New York

A gourmet cook is one who by simply reading a recipe can predict the outcome with fairly reasonable accuracy. Cooking is a creative outlet, and a gourmet cook has a natural bent for mastering the skill much like a skilled painter or accomplished musician has succeeded in their craft. A gourmet cook has an infectious enthusiasm, knowledge, and passion for food, cooking, and presentation. A gourmet cook is not afraid to experiment and to throw out what doesn't work. A gourmet cook responds to and is motivated by the comfort that cooking and creating bring.
—Nancy Guth, California

Chapter 2

The Cheapskate Gourmet Kitchen

A gourmet cook is a person with the ability and concern to prepare food from scratch that is tasty, zesty, and attractively presented.
—Alice Cook, Mississippi

If your kitchen is anything close to typical, it is likely furnished with a few pots and lids that don't necessarily match; a stack of baking and roasting pans that may or may not be the right size for the task at hand; several electric appliances, some of which don't work; a drawer crammed with utensils in a variety of conditions and configurations (some of which you don't know how to use but some day you might); several knives, none of which are sharp enough to be of much good; and at least one cookbook.

I believe the ideal gourmet kitchen should be furnished minimally. By that I mean it should contain an adequate supply of excellent quality, highly useful pieces of cookware and utensils.

If that doesn't describe your kitchen, don't give up on the idea of becoming a gourmet cook. Take inventory and dejunk your cupboards and drawers so that each piece of equipment you decide to retain is used often, performs adequately, and has its own place. That's the kind of simplicity that has a beauty all its own.

15

Following are several lists of kitchen equipment. The first is basic and necessary. The second lists items that are not mandatory but pieces you will eventually find needful as your gourmet confidence builds. If you don't already own things on the second list, don't drop everything and rush out to purchase them. You can add them to your equipment a bit at a time. Don't purchase hastily. The items you add to your kitchen from now on should be of the best quality you can afford because you'll likely have them for the rest of your life.

The third list contains items that spell pure luxury. Some of these things you may never need to own. Others you may want to have someday. Consider this a wish list. You'll have plenty of time to set aside the necessary funds, shop, and compare until you can select the brand and style that suits you perfectly.

List One: The Basic Equipment

baking sheets: Good flat baking sheets have many purposes other than baking cookies. At the minimum you should have one baking sheet without sides and one with sides all around that give the baking sheet a depth of about ⅜ inch. This sheet will work well for cream puffs and cookies but will also double as a jelly roll pan and other applications that require the contents be contained within the baking sheet.

biscuit cutter: These look like plain round cookie cutters but have very sharp bladelike edges and are used to cut biscuit dough, tart shells, filo dough, and wonton sheets.

bulb baster: Great for sucking up juices from the pan in order to baste; also works well for drawing off fat. A baster with a metal tube and rubber bulb are preferable to other kinds. Glass breaks easily and plastic melts.

cake pans: A pair of 8-inch rounds, 9-inch rounds, an 8- or 9-inch square pan, and a 9-inch by 13-inch (or similarly sized) rectangular pan. These can be either metal or glass and will be used for dessert and cornbread productions. (Always reduce the oven temperature by 25 degrees when using a glass pan to prevent the contents from sticking.)

cake racks: These are smallish racks that have little feet. They are used for cooling things like cookies, muffins, cakes, etc. Other applications can be as a meat rack when you do not want the roast sitting in the grease. You need one large or two small racks.

can opener: Yes, even gourmet cooks need to open a can now and again. A small manual model will work just fine.

cheesecloth: A very inexpensive product, this cloth will help you take that leap from ho-hum cook to gourmet all by itself. Cheesecloth is a very loosely woven cotton fabric that is used to cover turkey so that it keeps its juices and to tie together a bouquet of herbs and spices to cook in that soup, ragout, or in processing pickles. The little bundle is easily removed once the flavors have been incorporated into the treasure pot.

colander: This large "bowl" has many holes in the bottom to allow for draining and rinsing. Al dente pasta is transferred quickly to a colander to be rinsed under cold water to stop the cooking process, for instance.

cookware: This is the appropriate term for pots and pans. You need a 10-inch covered omelet/sauté pan (looks like a small skillet with a flat bottom; actually that's what it is, a small skillet or frying pan); 2½-quart covered saucepan; 4½-quart covered sauce pan; stockpot (a tall covered pot that can double to prepare pasta, boil potatoes, or prepare soup); large sauté pan (looks like a large frying pan with a large flat bottom and sides that are 2–3 inches high). Most kitchens have cookware in these approximate sizes. If what you have already is close or simply missing a few pieces, don't rush right out to make an uninformed purchase. Get by as best you can with what you have until you have educated yourself on cookware.

cutting board: You need a small wood or acrylic cutting board that can be stored in a cupboard or drawer.

Investing in Cookware

Here are some tips and hints to get you thinking about a possible future purchase of cookware. Because this will be an investment, become educated, move cautiously, and shop well. Prices vary greatly. In my opinion the top lines of cookware are Calphalon, All-Clad, and Analon. These are all highly regarded by the finest chefs in the world. Each of these brands comes with a lifetime guarantee and are backed 100 percent by their manufacturers. Of course there are many other lines of excellent cookware, some in the same price range as the big three. However, nothing seems to compare to these three when considering all categories, such as superior conductivity, even heating, and effective cooking surface. The use of aluminum and copper (which is the most conductive metal for cooking) in cookware is crucial. Each manufactures and produces different styles. Some are lined with anodized aluminum; others have the aluminum or copper bonded between layers of stainless steel.

Suggestion: Once you've narrowed your decision to one or two brands of cookware, visit your local housewares department or specialty cookware shop and ask to purchase a "preview pan" in the line(s) you are considering. For about $20 you can cook your little heart out and really decide what you like and what works for you. A $20 investment is a small price to pay when you consider you'll eventually spend upwards of $500 for an initial cookware starter set.

Now let me confuse you with yet another feature to consider. Should you buy nonstick or stainless? When the nonstick

Caution: When cutting meat (especially poultry) on a cutting board, one must be very careful to disinfect the surface. Bacteria can grow in the tiny grooves so that the next time you use it you end up transferring nasty bacteria to the new food. Make sure you clean your cutting boards with very hot

coatings were first introduced to the retail market in the 1960s, it had to be cared for with kid gloves. Even with the gentlest handling, eventually the nonstick surfaces chipped, scratched, or rubbed off, or worse, mixed in with the food. The techniques and nonstick products have been highly improved since their first introduction and are manufactured in such a way that the nonstick surface is integrated right into the pan, not just as a coating. Two features of nonstick to consider are that it is easier to clean than stainless, and if you don't like using a lot of oils in your cooking, nonstick is for you. Stainless of any quality will require the addition of oils when cooking most anything.

When all is said and done, the bottom line between nonstick and stainless cookware is personal preference. It's what you prefer in your cooking styles and tastes. Regardless of the type of cookware you use now or select for the future, never use metal utensils of any kind in your cookware. Never! Even though you may not be able to detect it with your naked eye, each time a metal utensil comes in contact with the metal surface, tiny scratches and crevices are being created. After time (a lifetime if you buy right) the surfaces will become uneven and irregular in finish, and that will affect your cooking. You'll have hot spots and ridges where bacteria and crud can hide. From this moment on break your metal utensil habit (don't get rid of them, however—they have other uses) and use only wooden, plastic, or rubber tools when stirring, whisking, flipping, and spearing in your cookware.

water and a kitchen-type disinfectant after each use.

flour sifter: In a pinch a large sieve or strainer can stand in as a flour sifter. However, these gadgets are readily available and very handy when preparing breads and desserts.

grater: A metal or plastic grater is used to grate hard things such as carrots, cheese, and nutmeg. Most graters have various-sized holes to produce either coarse or fine results.

knives: A good set of knives is heaven to a cook. Before feeling compelled to purchase new, consider what you already have. Chances are very good you have at least one knife that can be sharpened and serve you quite well for the time being. This and perhaps a smaller one or two will surely tide you over until you are in a position to make a serious knife purchase.

ladle: You will be thankful you have a ladle (looks like a cup on the end of a handle) when serving soups, ragouts, or filling pie shells and dessert bowls.

linens: You need about six good-quality heavy pot holders and/or oven mitts. An ample supply of 100 percent cotton dish towels is also necessary. Some should be large, woven cotton dish towels and a nice supply of smaller terry-cloth towels similar in size to bathroom hand towels. Many cooks enjoy the protection of an apron. Julia Child and Jeff Smith always wear a full apron with a small towel conveniently tucked into the wrap-around belt on which they continuously wipe their hands and mop up spills. One of your most important kitchen linens is a clean, white, all-cotton pillowcase. Yes, really!

loaf pan: You'll need at least one small rectangular pan (metal or glass) that has very high sides and looks like a small loaf of bread.

A Little Knife Advice

Here are some pointers to follow when you're ready to purchase. The best knives are high-carbon stainless steel, finely honed, and perfectly balanced, and again, expensive. But just like cookware, your knife investments will be a once-in-a-lifetime purchase. Diane Forley, French-trained chef/owner of the restaurant Verbena in New York City, says, "I think it's a mistake to spend a lot of money on a knife. It's more important to keep sharp whatever knife you do buy. You can get the best chef's knife but if you don't maintain it there's no point in buying it. A dull knife makes you work harder in cutting. And when a knife gets dull over time you can hurt yourself because you need to exert greater force to make it do its job."[1]

An excellent knife starter set that will handle all of your needs is a 3-inch straight-edge paring knife for peeling fruits and vegetables and cutting small items; a 5-inch utility (or sandwich) knife for slicing small items like cheese, fruits, or sandwich ingredients; an 8-inch chef's knife for slicing, chopping, and mincing; a honing device and a steel for maintaining your sharp edges between professional sharpenings. A long serrated knife is a luxury, and you'll be glad you have one when it comes to slicing crusty French bread, fresh tomatoes, or a prime rib roast because they have a gripping quality that allows one to slice paper-thin if necessary. Before investing in one, however, consider these facts about serrated knives: They stay sharp the longest, have very limited uses, and cannot be resharpened. Your kitchen knives should be professionally sharpened at a cutlery shop once every year or two and sharpened monthly (or more often depending upon frequency of use) at home for maintenance.

1. Regina Schrambling, "How to Stay Sharp in the Kitchen," *Good Housekeeping,* April 1996, 43–44.

How to Sharpen Knives at Home

In order to keep your knives sharp at all times, you need two things: a whetstone that sharpens the blade and a sharpening steel (a rigid metal rod that looks like a long, skinny sword on a knife handle) to straighten the blade. Look around for a sharpening device that includes a whetstone. Some knife sharpeners are constructed so that the knife blade is always layed to the whetstone at a twenty-degree angle. Some knife sharpening models have two fixed steels that allow you to swipe the knife through. Once sharp, swipe the knife at a twenty-degree angle along the steel (the same number of times on each side of the blade) to create a nice edge. If you cook every day, your knives should be maintained weekly. If occasionally, once a month is adequate.

Your knives should only be used on a cutting board. In my opinion wood makes the best cutting board because it's kinder to the blade than plastic. It is best to wash your knives by hand rather than putting them into the dishwasher. Chances of them smacking up against something (damaging the blade) or cutting into the interior of the dishwasher are great. Knives should be stored carefully between uses either by hanging individually or cradled in a wooden block specially designed to hold knives. Why? When they bang around in a drawer, metal against metal blades can become nicked and even bend. If you take care of your knives, they'll serve you well and make your cooking that much more enjoyable.

measuring cups: You need both wet and dry measuring cups. Here's the difference. Wet measures have more cup beyond the highest measurement, which keeps measured liquids precisely and makes it possible to transfer the liquid without spilling some of it. A dry measure's measurement line is at the very top. This way you can "dip" the cup into flour, for instance, and level it with a straight knife for a precise measurement. That would be impossible in a wet or liquid measuring cup. You need 1-cup, ½-cup, ⅓-cup and ¼-cup measurers in both wet and dry. I have a single wet measuring cup. It holds 2 cups maximum and has the line indicators for every possible amount of liquid down to ¼ cup. It works just fine for any application.

measuring spoons: You need a set that includes at the very minimum 1 tablespoon, 1 teaspoon, and ⅛ teaspoon sizes. From that basic combination you can precisely measure all different amounts. If you have a ¼-teaspoon and ½-teaspoon size, it will make things more convenient, but they are not mandatory.

mixing bowls: At least three of various sizes: one large, one medium, and one small bowl will serve all of your needs in the beginning. I prefer glass, earthenware, stainless steel, or copper, but if you only have plastic bowls, they will do for now.

muffin tins: These come in several sizes; however, the one with the most utility makes one dozen medium-sized muffins.

pastry brush: This looks just like a small paintbrush and is used to apply egg washes to fancy pastries, melted butter to bread, oil or grease to a pan in the preparation stage, and many other uses. Tip: You can either buy a "pastry brush" at a kitchen specialty store for five to six dollars, or stop into your home improvement center and purchase a small natural bristle paintbrush. Mine cost ninety-nine cents six years ago.

pepper/salt mills: The use of freshly ground pepper, coarse kosher salt, and other spices will become commonplace in your gourmet cooking.

pie pans: For sure you will need at least one 9-inch pie pan. If you intend to purchase, treat yourself to glass pie pans that are large and deep.

rolling pin: These rolling instruments are used mostly in the preparation of pastries, doughs, and breads. If you do not have a rolling pin, don't go out and buy something fancy. The best rolling pin I know of is a 2-foot length of 2- or 3-inch wood dowel available at any lumber yard or home improvement center. Raw wood must be seasoned (not sealed) before use. Rub in a generous amount of vegetable oil with a clean, soft cloth and allow it to season in a 150° oven for an hour or two.

rubber spatula: While these come in several sizes, the most common is about 2 inches wide at the rubber part. This is the one you really need; however, if you have other sizes, don't toss them out.

scissors: A pair of kitchen shears can be used for everything from cutting away poultry skin to finely cutting chives, scallions, and fresh herbs. "Kitchen shears" can be high priced in a kitchen specialty store; a suitable substitute can be picked up in a fabric store for a fraction of the cost, or better yet, clean up a pair you already own, sharpen the blades, and label it "Kitchen Use Only!"

strainer: A 3-inch strainer is extremely handy for draining berries, fruits, etc., and for rinsing small things that could easily jump down the drain. Also used for "sifting" confectioner's sugar over desserts.

thermometer: These come in two varieties. A meat thermometer, which is inserted into large cuts of meat, poultry, and wild game to determine the temperature at the center. A candy thermometer reports the temperature to much higher degrees than the meat thermometer and is used in making syrups, caramels, candies, etc. An absolute must since many of these items must be cooked within degrees of scorching.

timer: A reliable timer is a must in the gourmet's kitchen. If you rely on your eyes to tell you when something is done, you may be terribly disappointed from time to time. When purchasing this item, it is advisable to get a high-quality timer. It's well worth the money.

tongs: You'll need several pairs of tongs for lifting things out of boiling water, turning chops and cuts of meat, removing things from the oven, etc. A pair of salad tongs (big spoon and fork hooked together) is necessary if serving salad "family style."

utensils: A large cooking spatula (pancake turner), large regular spoon, a slotted spoon, a ladle, and a whisk. These should be made of reinforced nylon (looks like hard plastic) to prevent scratching of cooking surfaces.

wire whisks: A whisk is a wonderful tool you cannot be without. In fact, you really need two: one on the large side and a smaller one (not the miniature whisk that is used to mix cocktails). A wire whisk can be found in any kitchen specialty store, some groceries, and discount stores like Wal-Mart, Kmart, Target, Ikea, etc. A whisk has a long round handle out of which come big "loops" of rigid metal wire. Actually it looks like a teardrop-shaped birdcage. A whisk is used for stirring, mixing, and beating things like egg whites, sauces, cream, cakes, icings, and gravy. It is a miraculous invention because with little effort you can produce marvelous lump-free gravy,

Cheap Tip

The big round measuring lid from a container of liquid laundry detergent doubles as an adequate (and FREE) liquid measuring cup. Look inside and you will likely see marks indicating ¼-, ⅓-, and ½-cup measurements. Save a few of these big bottle lids because they also make dandy cookie cutters.

light and perfect meringue, and voluminous whipped cream.

wooden utensils: Three large wooden spoons in different sizes, a spatula, and cooking fork. Wooden utensils are often sold in sets and can also be purchased individually.

List Two

All of the items in List One plus:

coffeemaker: I'm very partial to the Bunn line of coffeemakers. They are workhorses and produce gallons of coffee without a complaint. The best feature is the reservoir, which keeps enough water for a full pot hot at all times. No waiting, ever. In fact, if you happen to pour in the cold water before the carafe is properly in place, you end up with a mess—the fresh coffee comes out that fast.

cookware: Once you're ready to expand your supplies and equipment to this list, it's probably time to start getting that good cookware.

electric blender: A blender makes puréeing soups, frappés, and popular health drinks wonderfully convenient and efficient. Not a must, but certainly a nice option.

electric mixer: In my opinion if you want to go for the best, hold out for a KitchenAid free-standing solid-state power mixer. You'll think you've died and gone to heaven. If this is too rich for your blood, a hand-held KitchenAid mixer will do just fine for almost all of the times you will need it.

food processor: A good processor can make your time in the kitchen more efficient. A good processor (my favorite is Cuisinart) will grate, chop, dice, and mix. To me it's my third and fourth hand. The time required to make pâté brisée or brioche is diminished by at least half without losing quality or taste. I guess you can tell I'm pretty crazy about my food processor.

ice cream scoop: In addition to scooping ice cream, a scoop is great for forming meatballs and scooping cookie dough.

knives: If you do not already have knives that you find perfectly heavenly, start looking. You've graduated to a more advanced level of gourmet, and now's the time.

mixing bowls: A good set of glass or earthenware mixing bowls will bring your kitchen skills to a new height. The heavy quality, impeccably smooth surfaces, and sound produced when whisking or mixing bring a delight to the soul.

parchment paper: Available in either sheets or rolls from a cake decorating or kitchen specialty store, parchment paper is unique and mandatory for the experienced cook. Wax paper, plastic film, or aluminum foil cannot substitute. Wax paper is flimsy, things stick to foil, and although plastic film is fine for covering foods for refrigeration, you don't want to cook with it. Parchment paper is used to line baking pans and cookie sheets and to wrap up fish for oven poaching.

salad spinner: Not very expensive, a salad spinner allows you to wash greens within minutes of actual dining and produce them cold, crisp, and dry. If you don't have one, don't buy one. Instead place the well-washed greens into a clean cotton pillowcase and step outside. Grasp the end of the case in one hand and spin it in a windmill-like motion next to your body. In about thirty seconds—just before your arm gets tired—the greens will be dry and the pillowcase will be damp. It looks a little silly, but it's incredibly efficient, especially when you are making large amounts of salad.

slow cooker: I find this to be a marvelous invention. I have a Crock-Pot, but many other brands basically do the same thing: cook food for a very long period of time at a very low temperature. The energy consumed is much less than using the oven for one-eighth of the time. It is safe to leave a slow cooker unattended, and it will turn out some pretty tasty dishes. Caution: It's easy to get into such a rut that everything, no matter how divergent, comes out of the slow cooker tasting the same.

springform pan: This is a delightful accessory for making cheesecake, tortes, and other desserts that have a molded quality. By releasing the spring, the side piece comes off and allows the dessert to be perfectly removed from the pan without turning it over, jiggling, melting in warm water, or trying to squeeze a spatula under the delicate confection.

stovetop kettle: There's nothing like a substantial, well-made kettle in which to boil water. If you already have one, you're way ahead of the game. If you have an electric kettle, that's passable, but in my opinion not as convenient for preparing tea, hot water for soups, gravies, etc.

Parchment Paper

Parchment paper has wonderful qualities that come in handy in the kitchen. First it has a high wet strength (making it essential for cooking *poisson en papillote*) and passes no flavor or chemicals to the things it touches. Food does not stick to parchment and releases quickly without a struggle. Professional cooks set cakes on parchment paper, bake cookies on it, line cake pans with it, make soufflé collars from it. Parchment paper can be found in cake decorating stores, bakeries, restaurant supply companies, and specialty kitchen stores.

toaster oven: A great little appliance for toasting bread, warming pastries, even baking potatoes. When cooking for two, you will find this to be a great energy saver.

List Three

Everything in Lists One and Two, plus the following pure culinary luxuries.

(Note: Depending on your culinary "bent," you may decide to add items to your personal List 3 that will enhance that specialty. For example, if you are drawn to Asian cooking, you will enjoy the many special utensils and wares unique to that particular type of cuisine.)

Following is a very brief and highly abbreviated wish list of some pieces of cooking equipment that may not be mandatory but certainly assist greatly. Just as in fine woodworking, the right tool for the right job makes the process much more enjoyable.

bread machine
clay cooker
espresso machine
fish poacher
ice cream maker
meat cleaver
mortar and pestle

pasta machine
pressure cooker
rice cooker
soufflé dishes
specialized baking pans
specialty graters

Food Staples for the Kitchen

Baking Staples:

baking soda
baking powder
cornstarch
flour (all-purpose)
sugar
confectioner's sugar
dark brown sugar

corn syrup
bread crumbs
Bisquick or Master Mix (see
   chapter 6)
nonfat dry milk
unsweetened cocoa powder
unsweetened baking chocolate

Seasonings/Herbs/Spices/Flavorings:

salt (kosher, sea salt, or table)
pepper
peppercorns (for the pepper mill)
pure vanilla extract (see chapter 6)
mint extract
almond extract
cinnamon
nutmeg
cloves
ginger
basil
oregano
chili powder
dry mustard
paprika
bouillon cubes (for emergency)
bay leaves
oils, vinegar, and other condiments
cooking oils (corn, safflower, canola)
olive oil
vinegar
solid vegetable shortening
nonstick vegetable cooking spray
mayonnaise
ketchup
soy sauce
Tabasco or other hot pepper sauce
Worcestershire or A.1. Steak Sauce
honey
mustard (Dijon-style)

Refrigerated and Frozen Staples:

milk
eggs
sweet butter
sour cream
cream cheese
large eggs
cheese (cheddar, swiss, monterey jack, parmesan, or romano)

Extra Virgin Olive Oil

This designation means this oil is the first oil cold-pressed from the best fruit of the olive tree—the natural juice of the olive. It's unmatched for freshness and flavor. The "extra" in extra virgin means premium or, simply, the best. Ordinary olive oil and light olive oil are refined with heat and chemicals after pressing to remove defects. Small amounts of virgin oil are added to restore some flavor and color.

Butter

The finest gourmet cooks always use unsalted butter (also called sweet butter) for a variety of reasons: When butter is salted during manufacturing, the cook loses control over the dish because the amount of salt can vary greatly from one brand to another and from one batch to another. Because salt is a natural preservative, salted butter lasts longer and is allowed a much longer shelf life in the market. Sweet butter, on the other hand, becomes rancid much more quickly, which means the shelf life in the market is much shorter. When you purchase sweet butter, you can be fairly certain that it is much fresher than the traditional, salted variety.

Produce Staples:
aromatics (onions, carrots, garlic, and celery)
potatoes

a variety of in-season fruits and vegetables

General:
white rice (not instant or minute)
raisins

tomato sauce
tomato paste

First Aid Supplies:[2]
One box or jar of dried onions
One box of grated parmesan cheese
One box of instant vanilla pudding

One can of cheese sauce or cheese soup
One can of clam chowder
One jar, bottle, or plastic lemon of reconstituted lemon juice

2. "First Aid Supplies" excerpted from *How to Repair Food,* copyright © 1987 by Marina and John Bear, used by permission of Ten Speed Press, P.O. Box 7123, Berkeley, CA 94707.

Two small cans or packages of hollandaise sauce
One box of mashed potato flakes
One large can of asparagus
One large can of pear or peach halves
Sour cream
One box of prepared baking mix (like Bisquick)
Two small cans of shrimp
One box of unflavored gelatin
One 12-ounce can of evaporated milk
Garlic powder
Flavored syrup

Note: Likely you have many of these first aid kit items on hand so buy the things you don't have and tuck them all away. They will come to your rescue on that fateful day when the meal you've planned has turned into the disaster of the century and the guests will arrive in just twenty-five minutes. See page 259 for "A Last Resort Dinner."

Here's what our panel of gourmet cooks had to answer when asked, "If you were stuck on that proverbial desert island, what cookbook, cooking gadget, utensil, and/or equipment would you just have to have?"

Food processor, wire whisk, rubber spatulas, cutting board, sharp knifes of different sizes, but especially my butcher knife and a paring knife.

—Jan Sandberg

Paradise Potpourri, *a wonderful cookbook prepared 20 years ago by the Pairs and Spares group of the St. Thomas Reformed Church, U.S. Virgin Islands. I have to strain through the "food and spatter" spots to read the recipes (I've never claimed to be a neat cook). My Henckel paring knife (to peel those potatoes I should have planted); of course, my Black & Decker power mixer; wire whisk for the roux I make from the broth of the fish prepared in my very old cast iron skillet; just in case I find an electrical outlet on this desert island, my Crock-Pot, Panasonic bread maker, and hopefully next year's Christmas present—a pasta maker.*

—Mary Ann Woirhaye

A vegetable steamer because steamed veggies add much more color and interesting texture to a meal.

—Patrick Schroeder

My food processor. I have a small "cheapy" one, but I'm looking forward to investing in a good one someday because I use it so much.

—Judy Bergman

Probably the New C! Good Housekeeping Cookbook *(copyright 1963) along with all my regional, ethnic, ingredient-specific, awards/contests, and celebrity chef books. Other items would be my Panasonic rice cooker/steamer, tongs, big spoon, cutting board, and favorite paring knife.*

—Marilyn McCormick

I cannot live without my Cuisinart (food processor). I'd be quite depressed without my mortar and pestle and completely joyless if my electric handheld pepper mill could not come along with me to this island.

—Nancy Guth

Chapter 3

$\mathcal{A}$ Crash Course
in Basic Technique

There's no doubt about it. The biggest drawback to excellent performance in the kitchen is an inadequate knowledge of the basics, those techniques one must master in order to turn out excellent dishes and meals consistently.

If there's a chapter of this book you might be tempted to skip, please don't let it be this one. Without a mastery of proper technique, your knowledge and desires aren't worth too much, and your chances of reaching a higher level of culinary excellence are slim at best.

I used to think kitchen technique consisted of stirring, folding, whipping, beating, and occasionally frappéing. (I learned the terms from the settings on my blender.) If the instructions called for anything else, I simply selected one of the above as a more-than-reasonable substitute. And if a little is good, more must be better, which meant ingredients, cooking times, and techniques. Amazingly, every once in a while I turned out something that was acceptable, and on a rare occasion I'd even hit the jackpot. But looking back, I realize it was pure luck—not something I could count on duplicating.

Hindsight is such a great vantage point. Clearly my lack of proper technique was responsible for rubbery meats, lead-heavy breads, tough pastries, more-gray-than-green vegetables, and mushy pasta. Cooking for me was something like playing the roulette wheel.

I've since learned it's not the price of the ingredients or complexity of the process that is responsible for the success of the final product. Rather, it's technical skill melded with precision and patience that makes the difference between a disaster and a delicacy.

You may be surprised how much your cooking techniques can be fine-tuned or simplified. Impeccable technique is achieved through knowledge plus practice, practice, and more practice. The reward of achieving technical excellence is the confidence you'll have in your ability to bring about success consistently. You'll no longer wonder if your bread dough will rise this time or flop again. You'll look forward to preparing gravy rather than leaving it to chance and hoping for the best. You'll be able to turn a bunch of plain broccoli into a gourmet delight by pairing it with your delicious homemade hollandaise sauce.

Some of the following techniques are simple and may be as commonplace to you as brushing your teeth. Other techniques are much more challenging and will take many practice sessions. That's OK! How long did it take you to learn to ride a bike or roller skate? How many years did you take piano or karate lessons? I think you get the point.

Basic Techniques

First of all, the most important "technique" is the art of following the recipe:

follow a recipe: The excellent cook knows how to read and follow a recipe and each instruction with all the precision of a brain surgeon because that cook knows that a good recipe works. It is a precise formula, not a suggestion. Failure in this area will keep you and your soufflés from falling flat on your faces. Here are the basic steps:

1. Assemble all ingredients before beginning.
2. Read all instructions before commencing.

3. Measure accurately. If you need 2 teaspoons of pure vanilla, don't grab a soup spoon to measure, justifying the action because it looks like about 2 teaspoons. Become a fanatic about precise liquid and dry ingredients.

4. Follow instructions to the letter. If you are told to mix certain dry ingredients in a separate bowl, do it. If partway through you must chill the dough for 30 minutes, do exactly that, and clean up the kitchen while you're waiting.

5. Know the language. If the instruction says to "cream the butter and sugar," find out what it means before you go on.

6. Respect exact temperatures. Make sure your oven is precisely calibrated.

7. The more advanced gourmet takes the freedom to amend and change a recipe.

bake: Baking, which uses a lower oven temperature than roasting, is used for gentle cooking of easily burned foods, especially those containing flour. Making sure the heat in the oven is even is crucial to the baking process. Often ovens that are used specifically for baking are equipped with stone or brick floors to collect and distribute the heat evenly. These ovens are also equipped with a mechanism that allows steam to enter at controlled intervals, for a controlled amount of time. This steam feature can be duplicated in home ovens by spraying cool water into the oven and quickly shutting the door, or by placing a pan of water on a rack below the baking item. Tip: If your oven has hot spots (places that seem to cook faster than others), you can avoid burning by changing the position of the food in the oven often and by using thicker or double-ply baking pans. To ensure even baking of cookies, simply invert an empty cookie sheet and place on the oven rack. Place the filled cookie sheet on top. This will guarantee even heating.

blanch: Blanching is one of the three cooking techniques that involves cooking food in or around water (the other methods are poaching and steaming). Blanching refers to a light and quick cooking of ingredients, most often in boiling water. Sometimes blanching is done in hot oil. Often blanching in boiling water is followed by shocking the ingredients quickly—dumping them into ice water, which preserves the crunch and color and stops the cooking process immediately.

braise: This is a low-temperature cooking technique in which food is cooked in a small amount of liquid in a closed container for a long time. This is an ideal method for cooking large cuts of tough meat and for vegetables that must be cooked thoroughly. Braising can also be used for cooking certain fish— those with firm texture that hold up to long cooking times. Braising helps to make tough meat tender by breaking down both kinds of connective tissue, collagen and elastin collagen, which is white and turns to gelatin and water when exposed to moist heat. Meat can also be tenderized by placing an acid, such as tomatoes or other acidic ingredients, in the braising liquid. Foods are most often browned before braising. Browning caramelizes any outside sugars, thus intensifying flavor, and helps to seal in the juices. After the braising liquid is added and the food is slowly cooked over a period of time, a rich liquid develops, which is often reduced and used as the sauce. The braising pan is usually oval or rectangular and fairly deep. A tight-fitting lid is a must, and solid handles make removing the pan from the oven much easier.

broil: Identical to grilling, except the source of heat comes from above the food placement.

calibrate oven: When your oven is set at 400°, you need confidence that that is the exact temperature inside the oven. You can check and calibrate your oven yourself. You'll need a good, reliable oven thermometer. Turn your oven on to 400°. Place your oven thermometer in the center of the oven and close the door. When the indicator light switches off, indicating that the selected temperature has been reached, immediately check the setting on the thermometer. If it is higher or lower than 400°, you must adjust the oven's thermostat. Look in your owner's manual for instructions. If you don't have one, call the manufacturer for instructions. If all else fails, experiment. My oven thermostat control is visible by removing the oven selection knob. Similar to a clock with an adjustment that indicates "faster" or "slower," my oven thermostat adjustment allows me to set it "hotter" or "cooler." It may take a few adjustments to get it just right.

clarify butter: Clarified butter is sweet butter from which the milk solids have been removed. To do so, put the butter into a large glass measuring cup in a warm (225°) oven and let it stand until it melts and the milky substance settles at the bottom. Place the container in the refrigerator until the butter hardens. Unmold the butter and scrape off the milky residue. Clarified butter will last almost indefinitely in a covered container that is stored in the refrigerator. Clarified butter is a main ingredient in hollandaise, béarnaise, and chron sauces; roux or beurre manié (a mixture of flour and butter used to thicken sauces and gravies; see chapter 8); and is excellent for sautéing because without the milk solids, clarified butter does not burn easily. The flavor of clarified butter is somewhat diminished when the milk solids are removed.

coat a baking sheet: There's nothing worse than baking beautiful cookies, pastries, or desserts only to have them hopelessly stuck to the pan once removed from the oven. Coating the baking sheet is an excellent way to prevent this kind of disaster. This technique can also be used in baking dishes, cake pans, and soufflé molds. First, generously rub sweet butter on the surface of the dish or pan, making sure to completely coat corners and sides as well as the horizontal surfaces. Liberally sprinkle sugar or flour (depending on whether the surface will be used for sweets or breads) on the buttered surface to form a coating. Shake the sheet or pan thoroughly in all directions so that all the butter becomes uniformly coated. Invert the sheet or pan over a waste container or the sink and give it a good whack to remove all excess flour or sugar. The coating should be light and uniform.

cream: Not a noun in this context, creaming is a verb referring to a technique used in baking desserts and cookies. To cream simply means to work one or more foods together until they are soft and blended. Generally the creaming process starts with butter. The sweet butter must be soft and at room temperature. If your butter is cold, do not force it by heating. Simply cut it into small pieces and allow to warm naturally. Typically you will be creaming sugar into the butter. You can do this by hand with a spoon or whisk or with an electric mixer. The speed should be moderate, and the creaming process should continue for a long time (probably 10 minutes or more) until the mixture is the palest of yellow and very light and airy.

cut in: This is a step in making pâté brisée and crumb toppings and can be done with a pastry blender or with two knives and a crisscross cutting action.

defrost: Because of health concerns, it is imperative that meat, chicken, fish, egg-based dishes, and casseroles containing any of those ingredients be allowed to defrost in the refrigerator. If you defrost these things in a microwave, cook them immediately upon being defrosted.

deglaze: After food is roasted, a glaze often forms in the bottom of the pan caused by high heat that has crystallized the sugars and juices in the food. This very concentrated glaze is used by the cook in a process called deglazing. When deglazing, the cook pours a room-temperature liquid, such as stock, into the hot sauté pan and scrapes loose the brown particles from the bottom of the pan, which creates a flavorful base for the sauce.

dredge: Often a recipe will instruct that the chicken or pork chops should be dredged in flour or some other type of dry ingredient. Simply place the dredging item into a shallow pan or bowl and press the item to be dredged into the mixture so that it becomes evenly coated on all sides.

eggs, beat: Sounds so simple, doesn't it? Don't be so sure. Beating eggs is a definite technique made up of several variations depending on what ingredients are involved with the egg beating. **Beating egg yolks and sugar.** When the instructions offer only recipe shorthand, "beat the egg yolks and sugar," this is the method you should follow. Begin by beating the yolks alone with an electric mixer or large wire whisk. You should use a bowl that is only slightly larger than your giant whisk for this reason: All of the egg mixture must be moving at the same time to achieve ideal results. Once you have the yolks moving pretty well, begin adding the sugar gradually—only a small bit at a time. In a while the sugar will dissolve into the egg. With each addition of sugar, the mixture will become a paler shade of yellow, and the volume will increase dramatically. Once all of the sugar has been added, continue beating until it reaches "ribbon stage"—when a bit of the mixture is allowed to drop down onto the mixture, it remains on the surface and looks like a piece of ribbon. **Beating whole eggs and sugar.** When the whites are included, you will be able to create greater volume. Whenever you are dealing with egg whites, it is important that your beating equipment be impeccably clean and free from any oil or grease, which will prevent the eggs from creating the greatest volume possible. A copper or stainless bowl is ideal, one that has a round bottom and is narrow and deep. Again you need to keep all of the product in motion at the same time. With your whisk or beater, blend the eggs and sugar in the bowl and proceed to set the bowl in a pan of almost-simmering water. Continue beating vigorously until the eggs are slightly warm to the touch (about four to five minutes) and the sugar is all dissolved. Remove the bowl from the simmering bath and continue beating for another ten minutes (or more) until the eggs are cool and form a thick, slowly dissolving ribbon. **Beating egg whites to peaks.** Stiff egg whites have a variety of uses. Basic meringue (stiffly beaten egg whites and sugar) is used in all kinds of desserts. It can be dried under a broiler high atop a pie; poached and called *oeufs à la neige;* when piped into a shell, basic egg whites and sugar become *vacherin;* mix with nuts and you have a *dacquoise.* Introduce fresh butter, and it becomes a classic butter cream. Preparing your

equipment for beating egg whites is very important. First the egg whites cannot contain even the
tiniest amount of egg yolk or fat. Even the cleanest
bowl and beaters should be prepared: Pour a tablespoon of vinegar and a teaspoon of salt into the
bowl. Mix it around with the beaters or whisk. Rub
the bowl and beater/whisk dry with a paper towel.
Do not rinse. The traces of vinegar and salt will
help stabilize the egg whites to ensure perfect
results. Place whites, which are at room temperature, in the bowl. Cold whites do not fluff well. Start
beating the whites at a slow speed until they
appear frothy, about two minutes. If you have not
rubbed the bowl with salt, add a pinch at this time
and ¼ teaspoon cream of tartar. Gradually increase
the beating speed through medium to high and
continue beating until you are able to form stiff
peaks that have a shine to them. If you are adding
sugar, begin doing so, one tablespoon at a time,
when soft peaks form. Continue beating until the
peaks are stiff. It is possible to overbeat egg whites,
so watch carefully and stop beating when those
shiny peaks begin to turn grainy.

fold in: This is a term used mostly in making desserts,
especially creams and meringues. The purpose is
to introduce and incorporate another ingredient
without destroying the airy or fluffy quality of the
finished mixture. For example, let's say we're folding meringue (a mixture of egg whites and sugar
that is whipped into billows of white froth) into
lemon curd. First mound the beaten egg whites on
top of the curd in a large bowl. Slide a wooden or
rubber spatula in a perpendicular position along
the surface of the meringue. Once you are almost
to the side of the bowl, turn the spatula one-
quarter turn, and cut down through the mixture to

the bottom of the container; turn again and cut across the bottom; turn a third time to cut up through the mixture on the opposite side so that you bring some lemon curd up and over the egg whites. You should be back where you started. With your opposite hand, turn the bowl a few times with each completed rotation of the spatula. Folding in should be done gently and minimally, only until the mixtures are slightly combined. Too much rigorous folding will quickly become stirring, and that will deflate the airy mixture.

fry: Frying is similar to sautéing, except when food is being fried, at least one half of the food is submerged in fat. There are two types of frying: deep-fat, wherein the food is completely submerged in oil, and pan-frying, when the food is only half submerged.

grill: This method of cooking requires that the food be placed over direct or indirect heat that is produced by a burning material (charcoal, wood) or a heating element. This is a very healthy cooking method, particularly for meat and poultry, because the internal fats tend to drip away during the cooking process.

hold knife for chopping: What I wouldn't give for an illustration right about now. Step 1. Comfortably grip your favorite chopping knife in your dominant hand of choice. Step 2. With your free hand hold the item(s) to be chopped securely on the cutting board. Move your fingers close to the location of the first cut and tuck your fingertips under. Step 3. Now rest the side of the knife blade against the middle section of your tucked-under fingers. The knife should become "glued" to this place on your fingers so that as you move your fingers back once the chopping has begun, the knife comes right along, making uniform results. Most of the time the knife will not completely leave the cutting surface. Instead, it should "rock" from the tip of the blade to the part closest to the handle without coming "unglued" from the tucked-under fingers. Now each downward motion makes another chop and encourages the tucked-under fingers to move back while bringing more of the item under the knife with those still-tucked fingers. This is a difficult technique to master, so start slowly and deliberately. And keep your eyes open, for goodness sake! I see no real value in chopping at the speed of light. Your speed will come all by itself as you become more proficient and confident. Practice on food items that are already destined for the garbage, like potato peelings, apple cores, etc. On a personal note, Martin Yan, the consummate expert on Chinese cooking, is my favorite chopper. He is very fast, precise, and never misses, even while wearing a blindfold. Good thing, too, because he chops with a large meat cleaver, the same type Julia Child uses to dismember chicken parts with one mighty blow.

knead: After the bread dough is thoroughly mixed, turn it out onto a lightly floured board or pastry cloth for kneading. Knead for about two minutes and then let the dough rest for about ten minutes. This allows the flour particles to absorb the liquids and facilitates kneading. To knead, fold the dough over on itself, then push it out with the heels of your hands. Give the dough a quarter-turn and repeat these two motions, using not just your arms but your whole body and setting a vigorous rhythm as you work. Knead for about ten minutes unless otherwise instructed. To test if the dough has been kneaded sufficiently, depress the dough with your fingers; if it springs back, it has been kneaded long enough.

measure flour: Whether the instructions of your recipe mention it or not, it is always best to use the following scoop-and-level method for the precise measuring of flour. A bit too much or not enough can mean the difference between a tough dough or one that's too wet, cookies that are dry as the Sahara Desert or run all over the baking sheet and onto the floor of the oven. Yuk. Plunge a dry measuring cup into a large container of flour and pull it out mounded high with flour. Using the straight edge of a knife, sweep off the excess so the flour is even with the top edge of the measure. If your instructions require that you first sift the flour, do so prior to measuring.

peel tomatoes: Peeled and seeded tomatoes are a staple ingredient in many recipes. Peeling raw tomatoes that will be presented in a garden salad is not necessary, but in my opinion, it is an added touch that subtly signals excellence. First remove stems and leafy tops from the tomatoes. Gently drop them into a pot of enough boiling water so they are fully submerged. Leave them in the boiling bath for about twenty seconds for fully ripened tomatoes, slightly longer if they are a bit green. Some of the skins may split at this point, which is a good sign but not mandatory. Transfer the blanched tomatoes to a bowl of ice water, and as soon as they are cool enough to handle, slip the skins off with the aid of your paring knife. Cut the peeled tomatoes into halves through the width, not through the stem. Gently press the flesh to remove all seeds. What remains is the tomato flesh and pulp. The skin and seeds can be added to a stock pot for another use. Alternate method for peeling tomatoes: Stick a fork into a raw tomato. Using the fork as a handle, gently roll it over an open flame (your gas range flame works well) until the skin is roasted, about twenty seconds. This roasted skin should peel off easily.

poach: Poaching food is achieved by placing food into a hot liquid and leaving it long enough to cook fully. Poaching liquid is not hotter than 180° and the poaching liquid is sometimes seasoned. Poaching liquid can be plain water, milk, water, with lemon, tomato, vinegar, or a stock plus aromatic vegetables and seasonings. Items most often poached are eggs and fish.

prepare garlic: Garlic cloves come neatly packaged in a group, called a head, held tightly together by a dry, white skin that forms a kind of chubby, teardrop-shaped vegetable. In order to get to the cloves, place the head of garlic on a cutting board in a diagonal position. Position it with one hand at the bottom and with the heel of your other hand crush it, which will separate the cloves while leaving them intact. Place one clove, rounded side up, on the cutting board. With the flat side of a heavy knife, whack the clove just enough to break the soft "shell" open. Remove the clove from the shell and cut off the root end. At this point you can mince the garlic clove using the purée chopping technique as follows: Lay the skinned clove on the chopping board. Place the flat side of the knife blade on the clove and smack it down and a bit forward with the heel of your other hand. This will mash it to a pulp. Now chop through the flattened clove until it is reduced to a uniform mass. Garlic is a unique seasoning. When the cloves are removed from the head but left whole in their skins, as many as three full heads (up to forty cloves) can be roasted and served with a chicken. The scent and taste will be barely noticeable, and your guests will enjoy eating the mild, sweet roasted garlic. On the other hand, a single clove can be puréed and added at the last minute to potatoes, vegetables, or salad. Just that much puréed garlic can permeate a whole room and stay on everyone's breath for a very long time. The same puréed garlic when added to a ragout and allowed to simmer for many hours loses most of its pungency and blends in with the other herbs and seasonings until it is hardly noticeable. Raw garlic chopped to a purée is garlic in its most powerful state.

roast: Roasting and baking are similar cooking techniques. Both rely on the use of radiant heat in an oven. Spit-roasting, the original roasting method, was used primarily to cook meats, fish, and fowl. Meat was skewered onto a large pole, then turned slowly over the open fire until roasted through. Oven roasting, the technique most often used today, is done in a hot oven with the food resting in a pan on the oven rack. Food is sometimes seared on top of the stove, then allowed to roast until the proper internal temperature is reached. Roasting food has its advantages because high heat is used, which tends to caramelize, producing a beautiful rich brown color and a complex, well-developed flavor. Roasting food also tends to require less attention than other types of cooking, such as sautéing. Any time food is roasted, it should be allowed to rest before serving so that the tissue can relax and the juices stabilize.

sauté: Sautéing is a cooking process in which ingredients are quickly cooked over moderate to high heat with a small amount of fat in a large, flat-bottomed pan. The word *sauté* comes from a French word *sauter*—a verb meaning "to jump." The technique is so named because a cook does not stir when sautéing food. While the pan is on the burner, the cook pulls it toward him/her with a rapid jerk. The food catches on the far lip of the pan, causing the food to jump in the air, thus rearranging the food without stirring. Because sautéing is a high-heat method of cooking, the fat used in the pan should not be one that burns easily. Fats that contain other solids will burn quickly; examples are butter, extra virgin olive oil, and nut oils. Fats that are heat resistant include most vegetable oils, corn oil, safflower oil, pure olive oil, and canola oil.

separate eggs: Many recipes call for only the white of the egg or just the yolk. It's unfortunate in these cases that whites and yolks come packaged together. However, separating them while leaving both intact is a technique easily mastered by anyone with two clean hands. Plan on spoiling a few eggs before you get the hang of it. Here are the two simplest techniques for separating eggs. Start with very cold eggs for the best results. Using the first technique, crack the raw egg on the side of a small bowl so that you hold one half of the shell in each hand. While keeping the yolk in one of the shells, allow the white to drip down into the bowl. Now transfer the yolk into the other shell so that more white can drop into the bowl. Keep transferring back and forth until as much white as possible is down in the bowl. Transfer the yolk (which by this time should be perfectly whole in one of the shells) into a separate container and discard the shells. If you should break a yolk, start again. A recipe calling for egg white only may be spoiled by the presence of even the tiniest amount of yolk. The second technique for separating eggs is a little messier but much more reliable. Crack the egg shell and pour its contents into your clean hand that is held over a small bowl. Allow the white to drip between your fingers into the bowl. With a little practice you'll learn to part with all of the white while retaining the intact separated yolk in your hand. Gently deliver it to a second small container.

steam: Steaming is a very gentle cooking technique and is different from blanching or poaching because the food sits above the water rather than directly in it. Steamed foods, because they are not placed in the water, retain their water soluble nutrients as well as most of the delicate flavors. Steam is produced at the point water boils (212° at sea level) and therefore is considered a low-temperature cooking technique. Steaming neither changes the color of food nor enriches its flavor; it produces vegetables that have *retained* their crunchiness, color, and flavor. A common way to steam is to fill a pot one-fourth full of liquid, usually water, then suspend a grid or perforated rack just above it onto which the food is placed. The liquid should be replenished as needed. It is important to cover the pan tightly when steaming and not to remove it until the end of cooking. By definition, steaming can take place in the oven. Cooking in parchment paper, such as with a piece of fish layered with herbs and vegetables, is also considered steaming because the fish steams in its own juices until cooked.

thicken liquids: Gravy, pudding, and sauces are all examples of items that are thickened to one degree or another. There are several thickening agents that will do nicely, depending on the type of liquid and thickness desired. Following are the standard thickening agents. *Roux:* Blend an equal amount of melted butter and flour and cook over low heat in a pan or pot large enough to hold your finished product. Stir constantly for two to three minutes. Pour the hot liquid to be thickened (stock, meat juices, etc.)

into the roux, while stirring vigorously. Continue stirring until the contents reach the boiling point. Make sure the liquid added is very hot, or you'll end up with disgusting lumps. *Beurre manié:* To thicken a soup or sauce that is finished but too thin, make a beurre manié by blending an equal amount of soft butter and flour with your fingers. Add to the boiling mixture a tiny bit at a time, stirring after each addition until the desired thickness is achieved. *Instant-blending flour:* This product, one brand of which is Gold Medal's Wondra, dissolves instantly in hot liquids without forming lumps. It should not be used in baking in place of flour. While this is a great product, it is very expensive. Other thickening agents costing much less are the classic thickeners of the serious cook. Cornstarch must be dissolved in cold water before it can be added to a hot liquid. Used a lot in Chinese cooking, this is the thickening agent that produces a translucent, shiny sheen to the gravy or sauce. Add the liquefied cornstarch a bit at a time to boiling liquid. Whisk constantly. Arrowroot is quite expensive and sometimes difficult to find. Similar to cornstarch in consistency and results, arrowroot is nearly tasteless and must be dissolved in cold water before its addition to hot liquids. Potato flour cooks quickly and smoothly in liquid, is transparent, and leaves no raw taste. Potato flour is especially nice in fruit and egg sauces but cannot be heated to more than 76°.

Chapter 4

Classic Cuisine-Speak: From Al Dente to Zester

I have a firm belief that if something is worth doing, it's worth doing well. I can think of no undertaking to which this principle applies more than to the fine art of food preparation. It costs nothing to know the correct term and then to use it appropriately.

Personally, I immediately respect someone's level of gourmet expertise when they demonstrate their respect for the art by using correctly pronounced words and terms.

Take Mary Ann Woirhaye, a gourmet cook you'll be hearing from in following chapters. It took only a few moments of reading her thoughts regarding this subject for me to mentally classify her as a gourmet with high standards and tremendous expertise. How? She used the proper terms when referring to ingredients and techniques. She has an excellent command of what I call classic cuisine-speak. She didn't say, "Make a basic white sauce." She said, "Prepare a classic béchamel." I'm not sure if I was more impressed with her "classiness" or with myself because I knew exactly what she meant. A snobbish attitude? I don't think so. It's simply a way of showing respect for the craft and presenting yourself as one who values excellence.

Here's the basic lingo you must know to classify yourself among serious gourmets. I suggest you set a goal over the next several months of memorizing each of the following terms and begin adding them one by one to your everyday vocabulary.

al dente: An Italian phrase that literally means "to the tooth" and is used as a test for doneness for vegetables or pasta and implies a condition that leaves a certain firmness, not soft or mushy. There's no good English word that conveys the exact meaning of *al dente*.

aromatics: Aromatics are vegetables like onions, shallots, leeks, garlic, carrots, and celery used primarily to lend their flavor and aroma to foods with which they are cooked. Sometimes they are simply dropped into the cooking pot, or sometimes a combination of chopped aromatics will provide a bed on which meats, fish, and poultry are braised.

arrowroot: A fine white powder or starch that comes from a tropical underground root. Arrowroot is used to thicken sauces and soups. Because it has no taste of its own and has remarkable clarity and appearance, gourmet cooks generally prefer it to cornstarch, which is used for the same purpose.

au gratin: Having a browned or crusted top made from fine bread crumbs as a result of being placed under a broiler. This term is often used to imply the use of grated or shredded cheese and/or a rich sauce or combination of ingredients that are served in the dish in which they are cooked.

au jus: Pan drippings or natural juices. An accompaniment made by straining juices from a roasting pan served without thickening.

bain-marie: A bain-marie or "water bath" is a container placed inside (or over) a second container filled with hot water. It is used to gently cook food by surrounding it with simmering water.

baking: Baking is a cooking method that uses low temperatures. Foods that contain flour must be handled at these lower temperatures. Such foods include pastries, breads, cakes, cookies, and pies.

balsamic vinegar: A barrel-aged vinegar, dark in color with a mellow, sweet/sour character, made from the *Trebbiano* grape in the region surrounding Modena, Italy.

basmati rice: A distinctively flavored, aromatic variety of long-grain rice. The individual grains are very small in size and are typically found in Indian and Pakistani cuisines.

béarnaise: A classical emulsion sauce (similar to hollandaise) made by combining egg yolks and a reduction of vinegar, shallots, and tarragon whisked together over low heat with the addition of butter and finished with chervil.

béchamel: A simple sauce made by combining a light *roux* (butter and flour cooked to a paste consistency) and milk. Béchamel is a basis for other sauces. With the addition of crayfish it becomes *Nantua*, with Gruyère cheese it becomes *Mornay*, and with onions it becomes *soubise*.

beurre manié: A smooth paste, made from equal parts of butter and flour, used to thicken sauces. Usually, it is whisked into boiling liquid a few small pieces at a time until well blended.

beurre noisette: Butter that has been gently heated in a sauté pan until it gives off a nuttylike aroma and turns golden brown in color. Often called "hazelnut butter" or "brown butter."

bisque: A thick, rich soup made with a crustacean or vegetable purée, classically thickened with rice and finished with cream.

blanch: A cooking technique where a raw ingredient is partially cooked for a brief period of time in boiling water or hot fat. As in a preparation technique, blanching tends to set colors and loosen skins and peels while sealing flavors.

blanquette: A creaming technique used for various dishes, the most famous being a blanquette of veal.

boil: A cooking technique where a raw ingredient is cooked in water (or other liquid) that is bubbling rapidly, as well as maintaining a constant temperature of 212° at sea level.

bombe: A layered, molded ice cream or frozen dessert, usually a half-sphere in shape, that is often decorated with whipped cream, nuts, and/or candied fruit.

braise: A cooking technique in which a raw ingredient is usually seared in fat and then tightly covered and cooked, partially submerged in a small amount of liquid over low heat for a long period of time.

brioche dough: A bread dough made light with eggs and rich with butter. Used in dessert-type breads and sweets such as cinnamon rolls.

broil: A cooking technique where a raw ingredient is cooked with radiant heat from above, usually with a gas flame or an electric element. Broiling is very similar to grilling, except the intense heat comes from above the food.

butter cream: A light and creamy uncooked icing made from butter blended with confectioner's sugar (or sugar syrup) and eggs. Occasionally a small amount of flavoring is added as well as a small amount of margarine or shortening for stabilization.

butterfly: The process of reducing a very thick piece of meat to a larger but thinner cut. With a sharp knife, simply cut the meat into two pieces through the thickest part on a horizontal plane. Stop cutting before you reach the other side, open the meat up through the cut and lay it out flat. It will resemble a butterfly and will cook much more quickly.

caramelization: The browning of natural sugars. This occurs between 320° and 360°. Vegetables, meats, and sugars can all be caramelized.

china cap: A cone-shaped, fine-meshed strainer with a handle usually made out of metal that allows liquid to pass through. Used for straining and puréeing foods. Also called a *chinois.*

chowder: A thick, hearty soup, made from a variety of ingredients, usually thickened with potatoes.

clarified butter: Butter from which the milk solids and water have been removed, leaving pure butterfat. Clarified butter has a higher smoking point but less butter flavor.

clarify: To make a liquid completely clear by removing all traces of fat and food particles. To clarify soup, for example.

compound butter: A mixture of raw butter and various flavoring ingredients such as minced herbs, lemon zest, or spices, creamed to a smooth consistency.

consommé: Rich, flavorful concentrated broth that has been clarified to make it clear and transparent.

crème fraîche: Heavy cream available in France that contains culture that allows it to ferment gently so it thickens like yogurt or sour cream. It can be boiled, reduced, and thickened without fear of curdling.

croutons: Small cubes of bread that have been dried out in the oven or fried, then seasoned. They are used as a garnish on salads and other side dishes. Homemade croutons have a fresh, delightful flavor that is preferable to the packaged variety.

crudités: Fresh, raw vegetables arranged in an attractive pattern with or without a dipping sauce.

cut in: To incorporate cold shortening (fat) into flour until it resembles coarse crumbs.

deep-fry: A cooking technique where a raw ingredient, usually coated with bread crumbs or batter, is completely submerged and cooked in hot fat.

deglaze: To swirl a small amount of liquid in a pan at moderate heat to dissolve cooked particles or caramelized drippings remaining on the bottom of a pan after sautéing or roasting.

degrease: To remove fat by lifting it off the surface of a cold dish or skimming it off the surface of a hot dish such as soup, stew, or sauces.

dice: To cut food into a uniformly small size.

dredge: To sprinkle with flour or sugar.

drippings: The accumulated bits of cooked matter and liquid left in a roasting pan after meat, poultry, or fish has been cooked. Use to make pan gravy.

dust: To sprinkle food lightly with dry ingredients, such as a dusting of confectioner's sugar on the top of a cake.

duxelles: Minced mushrooms that have been sautéd in butter until all their liquid has evaporated. This preserves them and condenses their flavor. They may be refrigerated or frozen in a tightly closed container and used, as needed, for seasoning.

egg wash: A mixture of eggs (yolks and/or whites) beaten with a pinch of salt and generally thinned with water or milk. Used to give shine to baked items or as an adhesive, such as when sealing the edges of ravioli together.

emulsion: A uniform mixture of two nonmixable liquids (usually oil and water) in which one is suspended within the other. Emulsions may be stabilized (or forced to not separate) with an egg or mustard and are classified as temporary, semipermanent, or permanent.

en papillote: A preparation technique in which raw ingredients are wrapped in parchment paper or aluminum foil and then cooked, causing the food to steam in its own moisture. A form of poaching.

fillet: As a verb, *fillet* means to remove bones from a piece of beef, chicken, or fish. As a noun, *fillet* means the food after the bones have been removed, as in fillet of sole or filet mignon.

fold in: A delicate scooping motion to combine a lighter mixture into a heavier one without deflating the final combination.

fricassee: To cook slowly, covered, over low heat until the resulting combination is extremely tender.

fry: Cooking a raw ingredient in hot fat over moderate heat.

garnish: Embellishing a dish as a way to finish it and make it look appealing and attractive.

gazpacho: A cold Spanish soup, traditionally made from chopped or puréed raw vegetables.

glaze: To apply a coating on the surface of certain foods to give them a shiny or smooth appearance.

gluten: A sticky protein substance that remains when starch is washed out of flour.

grill: A cooking technique in which a raw ingredient is placed on an open grid and exposed to intense heat from underneath. This is a healthy way to cook because much of the fat drips away during the grilling process.

grind: To reduce food to tiny particles either by hand (chopping) or in a food grinder or food processor.

hard-crack stage: A condition registering 300° to 310° on a candy thermometer, in which a drop of boiling sugar syrup shatters into hard, brittle threads when immersed in cold water.

herb bouquet: This is a combination of herbs (a small traditional bouquet would include four parsley sprigs, a small bay leaf, and ¼ teaspoon thyme but might include garlic, savory, or oregano and spices such as cloves or juniper) which are bundled together and tied in cheesecloth. The *herb bouquet* or bouquet garnish is dropped into a variety of dishes, such as soup, stew, roasts, etc., and removed prior to serving. This eliminates the need for straining the liquids.

herb butter: Sweet unsalted butter into which fresh herbs such as parsley, dill, chervil, or tarragon are blended.

hollandaise: One of the five primary sauces. A classic emulsion sauce made from a vinegar reduction, clarified butter, and egg yolks, flavored with lemon juice.

infused oil: A seasoned oil made by combining a light oil with a flavoring agent such as blanched, puréed herbs or spices, sometimes done over heat.

Italian meringue: A dense, hot meringue made by gradually pouring a boiling sugar syrup (250°) slowly into partially beaten egg whites, which is then beaten to a stiff-peak consistency.

julienne: An ingredient is cut into very thin sticks approximately ⅛ inch by ⅛ inch by 1 to 2 inches long. Usually, a descriptive term for vegetables.

knead: To work dough by pressing and stretching it with the hands. Kneading is a manual process that blends all the ingredients in bread dough so that the yeast is distributed evenly. Kneading also gives the dough elasticity and a smooth, even texture.

marinate: To cover food, such as meat, fish, and chicken, with a seasoned liquid and allow it to remain for several hours or overnight to render it more flavorful and tender.

mayonnaise: A cold emulsion sauce made from oil and vinegar emulsified with egg yolk. Considered one of the foremost cold sauces.

melon baller: A small hand tool whose curved, cup-shaped blade is used for cutting fruits, vegetables, and other soft-fleshed foods into balls. Also called a *Parisienne scoop.*

mince: Chopping an ingredient into very fine pieces.

pan fry: Cooking a raw ingredient over moderate heat in a liberal amount of fat in an uncovered pan. Similar

	to frying.
parboil:	To precook food in boiling water for a very short time.
parchment paper:	Nonwaxed, moisture and heat-resistant baking paper, sold in sheets or rolls, that is used for many culinary purposes. Examples: cooking in parchment (*en papillote*), making small piping bags, and lining baking sheets.
pare:	To remove the outer skin of fruits and vegetables.
pastry bag:	A soft, pliable canvas, plastic, or nylon bag opened at both ends, often sold with a selection of numbered plain or star-shaped metal tips, used to pipe fillings, puréed foods, or icings.
pinch:	The amount of an herb, spice, or seasoning that can be picked up between the thumb and forefinger.
pipe:	To force a stiff mixture through a pastry bag fitted with a metal tip to make a decorative border or filling.
pipérade:	A colorful garnish of sliced onions, green and red peppers, and garlic sautéed in olive oil.
pith:	The white fibrous skin immediately under the outer skin on certain fruits and vegetables, notably citrus fruits. The pith of lemons, limes, grapefruits, and oranges contains high amounts of bitter and unpleasant-tasting oil.
poach:	A cooking technique wherein raw ingredients are cooked very gently in simmering water or other liquid (about 160° to 180°). Poaching is a slower cooking process than blanching. Many times the poaching liquid (water, broth, milk) is well seasoned. Some types of fish can be poached in an aromatic liquid. Eggs are poached in clear, unseasoned water.
primary sauces:	The five basic sauces most often used in the production of secondary sauces: béchamel, velouté, sauce espagnole (also called brown sauce), tomato

sauce, and hollandaise.

proof: To test yeast for potency; to ensure it is still active or alive.

provençale: The literal translation is "with tomatoes, garlic, and olive oil," and sometimes olives.

purée: A preparation technique in which a food has been finely mashed and/or strained to a thick, smooth pulplike consistency. Name used to describe food prepared in this manner.

ragout: A stew simmered in liquid. Same as fricassee.

reduce: To boil down a liquid to decrease its volume and increase its flavor.

relish: A well-seasoned mixture of chopped vegetables and/or fruits, often preserved with sugar and/or vinegar, used as an accompaniment or garnish to offer contrast of flavors and texture to a plate.

render: To make solid fat liquid by heating it slowly.

ribbon stage: Describes a stage where ingredients—typically eggs and sugar—have been beaten together to a certain consistency. A mixture is thick, pale yellow in color, and forms a ribbonlike design when it is lifted and allowed to fall back into the bowl.

roast: A cooking technique in which a raw ingredient is cooked surrounded by hot, dry air in an oven or on a spit over an open fire. The high heat causes foods to caramelize, which adds a beautiful rich brown color and a unique flavor (not to be confused with burning).

roux: A pastelike mixture of equal parts of flour and a fat (usually butter) cooked to varying stages and used to thicken liquids. The length of cooking time determines the color and flavor of a roux. Roux can be white, pale blonde, or brown. A light roux is used for making light soups as well as for cream and white sauces, while a dark roux is used for making dark-colored soups and heavier sauces.

sachet: A bag of spices and aromatic fresh herbs, tied

together in a cheesecloth bundle, that is used for flavoring a stock or sauce. A typical sachet contains parsley stems, cracked peppercorns, dried thyme, and a bay leaf.

sauté: A cooking technique in which raw ingredients are quickly cooked in a small amount of fat in a large, flat-bottomed pan. Comes from the French word *sauter,* meaning "to jump." The proper technique is described in chapter 3.

scald: Heating liquid to just below the boiling point (180° to 190°).

score: To make steam holes or vents in pastry so the steam will escape and keep the inside from becoming soggy.

sear: To cook meat rapidly over high heat to seal in its juices and flavor.

simmer: Cooking a raw ingredient in water (or other liquid) over low heat while bubbling slowly, as well as maintaining a temperature just below boiling, about 185°.

simple sugar: A sugar syrup made by combining water, granulated sugar, and light corn syrup, cooked over low heat until clear and then boiled until desired concentration is reached.

soft-ball stage: A condition registering 234° to 240° on a candy thermometer, in which a drop of boiling sugar syrup forms a soft, pliable ball when immersed in cold water.

soft-crack stage: A condition registering 270° to 290° on a candy thermometer, in which a drop of boiling sugar syrup forms firm, pliable threads when immersed in cold water.

sorbet: A frozen flavored ice, usually made from fruit juice/and or purée, that is similar to ice cream but does not contain any fat or egg yolk.

soufflé: A basic soufflé is a white sauce (béchamel)

enriched with egg yolks and cheese, into which beaten egg whites are folded.

steam: A cooking technique in which raw ingredients are cooked directly or indirectly by the steam created from boiling water or other liquids. Perhaps the best method of retaining a food's natural texture, shape, flavor, and vitamin and mineral content.

steep: To pour boiling water or other liquid over food and let it sit in the liquid.

stew: A cooking technique similar to braising. Raw ingredients are browned, covered with a liquid, and then simmered.

stock: The aromatic liquid left over from cooking meat, poultry, or fish with herbs and vegetables.

sweat: Cooking a raw ingredient in a small amount of fat over low to medium heat without caramelization/color until it softens and releases moisture.

temper: Two ingredients, each with different temperatures, are successfully combined. By adding small amounts of the hotter ingredient to the cooler one, you begin to balance their temperatures before folding them together.

thickening agents: An ingredient that when added to a liquid causes it to thicken. Such common gourmet agents include flour, beurre manié, instant-blending flour (an example is Wondra), cornstarch, arrowroot, and potato flour.

timbale: Any food (chopped or puréed cooked vegetables, chicken livers, or ham) baked with eggs and seasonings in a deep dish or mold.

truss: To tie a chicken, turkey, or roast with string so that it keeps its shape during cooking.

zest: The colored and outside fragrant portion of citrus fruit. Remove the zest for use in a recipe by gently stripping or grating the orange, lemon, or lime, making sure to remove only the colored portion;

not the pith (the white between the peel and the fruit), which is very bitter.

zester: Small hand tool used for removing the colored portion of citrus peel in thin strips.

Chapter 5

To Everything There Is a Seasoning

Nothing in the kitchen is more intimidating to the unskilled cook than a cupboard full of herbs and spices and a recipe that simply instructs, "season to taste," or "taste and correct seasoning as needed."

It's time to disarm any fears of the unknown, to establish a simple list of must-haves for the basic gourmet kitchen, and to help you understand the basic use and purpose of the most-often used herbs and spices. This knowledge will provide you with comfort and confidence to make use of nature's miraculous multipurpose plants.

Definitions

Herb: A seed plant, the aboveground parts of which die at the end of each season. Some herbs have medicinal properties; others are used as food or seasoning and are called culinary herbs or potherbs.

Spice: Aromatic flavorings made from parts of plants. The term *spice* is usually applied to pungent plant products, especially plants native to tropical Asia and Moluccas, the Spice Islands or Indonesia. The term *spice* often includes herbs that are the fragrant leaves of herbaceous plants.

You can see that there is not a clear-cut differentiation between herbs and spices. All herbs are spices, but not all spices are herbs. In the final analysis, exact and precise definitions of *spices* and *herbs* don't really matter. What matters is your success and pleasure in utilizing nature's gifts of herbs and spices.

◆ **Basic Rule #1:** Herbs and spices should never overwhelm. The purpose of any seasoning is to provide a subtle accent, an enhancement to the natural flavors.

◆ **Basic Rule #2:** It takes three times as much fresh herbs to give the same flavoring of one amount of dried herbs.

◆ **Basic Rule #3:** There are rules about which herbs to use. The decision of what herbs should be introduced with what dishes and how much, is in your hands—or rather, your taste buds.

Herbs

General Guidelines

If the taste is new to you, start by adding a small amount; you can always add more, but you can't take it out.

Note that some herbs lose their flavor quickly when they are subjected to heat and should be added near the end of the cooking process.

When you add an herb to something you're cooking, you should "bruise" the herb first to release the oils that give it the flavor. If it's a dried herb, crumble it into the pot. If fresh, tear or mash with the back of a spoon first.

Don't hold the jar right over the saucepan while you pour out the herb. Steam from the pan will get into the jar and be absorbed by the herbs.

Even though it seems convenient, don't store herbs right over the stove; heat is bad for them, and that means direct sunlight too. The best storage place is in a cool, dark cupboard.

Dried herbs lose most of their flavor after a year. This is one advantage to growing your own—you know exactly how old they are.

There's been a lot written and reported about the safety and propriety of some herbs in recent years. Some exotic herbs have become controversial, especially in the world of medicine. The herbs and spices we'll cover in this chapter are items you would buy from some source, either a manufacturer of commercial seasonings, grocery store, greenhouse, or seed company—not plants growing in the wild.

basil: In 1992, herb growers who supply fresh herbs to restaurants and supermarkets reported that their most requested herb, by a long shot, was basil. Basil is most often used to enhance the flavor of tomato-based foods. It adds exquisite flavor to fresh tomato salads, tomato sauces, spaghetti sauce, pesto, minestrone soup, zucchini, lamb, omelets, and scrambled eggs. Basil has a medium flavor. Dry basil can never approach the goodness of fresh basil; however, never hesitate using dry when fresh is not available.

bay: Mostly used in the form of single leaves, there is a great difference between the California and Mediterranean varieties of bay. Experts agree that imported (Mediterranean) bay is far more desirable, but if you have California bay, use it with great care because it has a much stronger flavor. Bay leaf is essential in a bouquet garni (to follow), and something doesn't seem quite right if a pot roast or pâté isn't cooked with a bay leaf. Bay leaf is always removed prior to serving. Bay leaf is most often used in soups, stews, spaghetti sauce, and other dishes that are subjected to long simmering. Excellent in marinades for poultry and meat. Very strong flavor.

chervil: Fresh chervil looks very much like parsley, and of the most common herbs, chervil loses the most flavor when dried. In French cuisine, chervil is considered one of the finest herbs. Chervil works well in omelets and other egg dishes, with chicken and veal, in sauces and light soups. Chervil should always be added at the end of the cooking process. Mild flavor.

chives: Chives, a member of the onion family, are preferable in their fresh state. If not available, select freeze-dried before frozen. Chives should always present a definite green color, not brown, and should be added at the end of the cooking process. Best when added to cream soups and sauces, in omelets, topping baked potatoes, cottage cheese, and cream cheese. Mild flavor.

cilantro or coriander: The seeds of these herbs are referred to as coriander; the leaves, cilantro or Chinese parsley. The leaves and the seeds are used quite differently and are not interchangeable. Ground coriander seeds are sometimes used in baking, whole seeds in pickling and preparing aromatic vegetables. Cilantro leaves have a unique and strong flavor and are used most frequently in Mexican, Indian, and Chinese cooking. Strong flavor.

dill: In its fresh state it is called dill; dried, it becomes dillweed. Dill seed is most often used in pickling. Fresh dill is good with fish and cucumbers and is basic to Scandinavian and Russian cooking. Even though dill has a lovely flavor, it should not be overdone. Medium flavor.

marjoram: This herb has a very pungent and strong flavor when fresh. Dried marjoram is much milder and loses its flavor quickly. Marjoram is excellent with grilled fish, egg dishes, chicken, pork, lamb, hamburgers, meat loaf, carrots, peas, potatoes, tomato dishes, and especially with summer squash. Medium flavor.

mint: Dried mint is OK; fresh is much better. Quite prolific in temperate climates, this is an herb that when allowed to roam freely can take over an entire yard. The most popular use for fresh mint is as a garnish for iced tea and other cold drinks. Other excellent uses include fruit salad; cooked with peas, carrots, potatoes, and zucchini; sauce for lamb; yogurt-based sauces; and soups. Medium flavor.

oregano: Dried oregano is much more pungent than fresh. Dried oregano should be used up and not stored long. Once it changes color, it loses its character and tastes stale. Mostly used in spaghetti sauce, pizza, and other Italian dishes; meat loaf, hearty soups, and casseroles. Strong flavor.

parsley: There's probably no good excuse for purchasing dried parsley since fresh is so prolific and available year round in the produce section of every grocery store. Dried parsley flakes are tasteless and used more for a pleasing visual effect. Fresh parsley is a seasoning that brings out other flavors in a dish. Curly parsley is tasty and decorative; Italian parsley has a flat leaf and a more pronounced flavor. When fresh chopped parsley is rubbed with other dried herbs it is surprising how the herbs seem to come to life. Fresh parsley is used in soups, stews, and casseroles, with omelets and scrambled eggs, with boiled potatoes and potato salad, and in green salads. Medium flavor.

rosemary: This herb is very pungent both fresh and dried. Best with all kinds of meat, especially lamb, pork, chicken, and stuffing for turkey, biscuits, breads, carrots, beans, and winter squash. Strong flavor.

savory: Summer savory is the most common and very versatile—all-purpose for most American dishes. Summer savory is the number one herb for beans. Also used in lentil soup, meat loaf, vegetable soup, deviled eggs, potatoes, and tomatoes. Winter savory is a perennial plant with a very strong flavor and limited uses. Strong flavor.

tarragon: This is a beautiful herb that has a delicate, subtle, lemon-and-licorice flavor. Especially good in dishes where flavors do not compete, like eggs, chicken, fish, veal, omelets, scrambled eggs, béarnaise sauce, and herbal vinegar. Add at end of cooking. Strong flavor.

thyme: This herb is very strong and essential to a bouquet garni, beef stew, pot roast, hearty soups, clam chowder, chicken, fish, and many vegetables.

Herb Blends

In many recipes and articles about cooking, references are made to herb combinations, such as *fines herbes, bouquet garni,* and *ravigote.* Of course the novice cook would either omit these foreign ingredients, assuming they can't be that important (and end up with a bland dish), or skip the recipe altogether, figuring they must represent some exotic and unachievable gourmet reference. While the following herb blends are common combinations for French recipes, they are simply combinations of herbs that taste good together.

fines herbes: Chervil, chives, and one of these: tarragon, thyme, marjoram, or basil. The chosen herbs are chopped very finely (thus *fines*) and added at the end of cooking.

bouquet garni: This refers to a combination of herbs (often spices too) that are bundled together in a piece of cheesecloth, tied with a piece of string, and added to the dish while it is cooking. This allows for easy and complete removal of the bouquet prior to serving. Typically, these fresh herbs are used in a bouquet garni: bay leaf, thyme, and either parsley or chervil.

herbes de Provence: A traditional French blend of basil, thyme, savory, fennel, and lavender flowers.

ravigote: A blend of herbs used to create a French sauce that is also called *ravigote:* parsley, tarragon, chervil, and sometimes chives.

a lovely herb blend: 2 parts marjoram, 2 parts savory, 1 part basil, 1 part thyme, 1 part tarragon. This is an all-purpose blend for many meat and vegetable dishes.

another lovely herb blend: 2 parts basil, 2 parts thyme, 2 parts parsley, 1 part grated lemon peel, dried. This blend is excellent on chicken, fish, and many vegetables.

bouquet garni for fish: 2 tablespoons celery leaves, 2 tablespoons dried parsley, 2 bay leaves (broken into pieces), 1 teaspoon dried basil, ½ teaspoon dried sage, ½ teaspoon dried savory, ½ teaspoon fennel seed. Mix all ingredients, divide into three equal portions, and tie into cheesecloth bags.

bouquet garni for beef stock: 2 tablespoons dried parsley, 2 tablespoons dried celery leaves (or lovage, which has a celery taste), 2 bay leaves (crumbled), 1 teaspoon dried marjoram, 1 teaspoon dried thyme, ½ teaspoon dried savory, ¼ teaspoon dried sage, powdered. This makes enough for three garni bags.

salad dressing blend: 1 tablespoon dried marjoram, 2 teaspoons dried thyme, 2 teaspoons dried savory, 2 teaspoons dried basil, 1 teaspoon dried sage. Use electric blender to mix all ingredients thoroughly; store in covered jar. To make salad dressing, combine 2 teaspoons of blend with ¾ cup salad oil and ⅓ cup vinegar. Also good on cooked vegetables and fish.

herb blend for chicken: 1 tablespoon dried thyme, 1 tablespoon dried marjoram, 2 teaspoons dried rosemary, 1 teaspoon dried sage.

herb blend for beef: 1 tablespoon dried marjoram, 1 tablespoon dried thyme, 1 tablespoon dried basil, 1 teaspoon celery seed. Use in meat loaf, hamburgers, or pot roast.

When it comes to herbs, the best rule of thumb is to use the freshest available. There was a time when herbs could only be purchased in a can from the store or grown on your farm. Now, however, fresh herbs are usually available in the typical local grocery store. But the most convenient way to have the very freshest all the time is to grow your own. Herbs can be successfully grown in a small garden, in patio containers, or right on your windowsill.

If you are certain that you'll never grow your own herbs and can't be bothered with frequently purchasing fresh ones, no problem. Just follow these guidelines when buying, storing, and using dried herbs:

◆ Store in the refrigerator or in a dark, dry cupboard.
◆ Discard after one year (write date of purchase on the container).
◆ Crush dried herbs between palms of hands before adding to the dish.
◆ Never hold a dried herb container over a hot pot (moisture from the steam affects the jar of herbs).
◆ Most recipes assume the herbs required will be dried. If using fresh, multiply the dried amount by three for a proper fresh conversion.

Growing Herbs

Herbs are incredibly easy to grow. Start with plants, not seeds, for your first garden. Small herb seedlings are available in the nursery section of any home center or commercial nursery. If detailed written instructions for the care and maintenance of the plants are not included, check with the salesperson. The best place to plant is a sunny, well-drained area. Raised beds provide the best drainage, as herbs don't do well in wet, low areas.

If you don't have room for an herb garden in the ground, grow one in pots, either outside on your patio or on a sunny windowsill. Also, if your winters are miserable, you can still have fresh herbs year-round. Grow herbs in shallow pots during the winter months and transfer to the great outdoors during the growing season.

Fortunately herbs are neither temperamental nor fragile. They don't need constant watering or fertilizing, and bugs don't really like them because they give off potent smells that seem to repel the little critters. You don't really need a green thumb to farm herbs. Any color will do!

Harvesting Herbs

Rather than harvesting the amount of herb you need at the moment, try to plan ahead and cut what you need in the morning—after the dew has dried, but before the sun is hot.

Drying fresh herbs should be done in a spot where air circulates thoroughly (usually upside down or lying flat on an open-air rack) out of direct sunlight. When completely dried, strip the leaves from the stem. To be on the safe side, put dried herbs in a 200° oven for ten minutes. This kills any insect eggs that happen to be in with the leaves. Now you're ready to store.

A little known fact is that fresh herbs freeze really well. Put fresh, cleaned, and dried (completely free from water) herbs on a tray in the freezer for a few hours. Once the herbs are frozen, put in freezer bags for long-term storage.

Remember that when using fresh herbs you need to release the herb's fragrance by bruising them with the back of a spoon or with your mortar and pestle.

Tip: If you have an overabundance of fresh herbs, try storing them by making herb butters, which can be frozen and used during winter months on homemade bread, melted over vegetables, or swirled in a simple sauce to provide a great burst of summer flavor. To make herb butters, chop a cup or more of fresh herbs with a stick of softened butter and blend until smooth. Add a few drops of lemon juice.

Spices

One of the simplest ways to boost flavor and improve your cooking is to toss out stale jars of dried ground spices (the typical shelf life of these ground spices is one year) and to buy whole spices to grind yourself. Heating a spice, whether toasting it dry or frying it in a bit of oil, further enhances its flavor, giving the spice a fuller character.

Whole spices have four times the shelf life of ground spices because their seed coatings and barks protect their flavors, which aren't released until they are ground or heated. A coffee grinder devoted to spice makes grinding a snap, though you can also grind spice, especially small quantities, in a mortar and pestle.

allspice: Allspice is a distinct spice, not a collection of spices as the name might imply. Allspice is used mostly in baking and in pâtés and terrines.

anise: While anise comes both in seeds and ground, the ground version is typically assumed in most recipes unless otherwise indicated. Anise has a delightful and strong licorice flavor and is an ingredient mostly called for in cookies.

cardamom: A spice that is bought whole or ground (rather pricey, I might add) and is used in baking.

chili powder: Made from chilies that have been dried. Commercial chili powder is only mildly hot. Ground chili is usually labeled "hot" and should be used with caution.

cinnamon: Ground cinnamon is used in desserts, main dishes, and drinks. Mixed with granulated sugar, cinnamon is wonderful on French toast or pancakes or sprinkled on a crisp slice of apple. Stick cinnamon is used primarily in mulled winter drinks and in sugar syrups for preserving.

cloves: Ground cloves are used in baking. A few whole cloves, stuck into an onion or tied in a cheesecloth bag, often lend flavor to soups or stews; press them in a scored ham to bake.

curry: Curry is a blend of turmeric, cumin, coriander, fenugreek, red peppers, and other strong spices. It originated in the cooking of India and should be used sparingly. Curry is often used to accent sauces or eggs. Curry varies greatly in composition from one brand to another, so the best rule of thumb is to purchase only a good, reliable blend of excellent quality.

fennel: Fennel seeds have a licoricelike flavor and should be used judiciously, or the flavor will turn bitter. The bulb of the fennel plant is much like celery and can be chopped raw and added to salads. Fennel is one of the essential aromatic vegetables.

ginger: Ground ginger is used primarily in baking; candied ginger is used in desserts. Fresh ginger root is common in Chinese cooking and has become a staple in the produce section of most grocery markets. Refrigerated, fresh ginger will keep for about a week. Kept in the freezer, ginger will remain usable longer. To use, simply cut off the amount you need at the moment and return what's left to the freezer.

mace: Mace, the outside covering of nutmeg, comes dried and ground. Mace has a much milder and lighter flavor than the nutmeg it encases and is classic with pound cake. Mace is typically required in baking and desserts.

mustard: Dry ground mustard is made of finely ground mustard seeds; it's very strong, so use mustard in small quantities. Prepared mustards are not the same as mustard seeds and, unless specified differently, if the recipe calls for mustard, it means mustard seeds.

nutmeg: Ground nutmeg loses its flavor very quickly. It is advisable to purchase whole nutmeg and grate it fresh (using the smallest holes on your grater) as needed. Only a few gratings give a fragrant taste to certain vegetables, egg dishes, and sauces; however, nutmeg is used mostly in desserts.

paprika: Many paprikas are more color than flavor, so it's advisable to purchase imported Hungarian paprika. Most dishes call for sweet paprika rather than the hot variety.

pepper: The best way to achieve the brightest and most vivacious flavor is to grind whole peppercorns as needed.

pickling spice: This is a mixture of whole spices such as coriander, mustard seed, cinnamon, bay leaves, allspice, dill seed, ginger, cloves, and peppers, and is used exclusively when making pickles.

poppy seeds: Most often used in rolls and other baked products, poppy seeds are also good tossed with noodles and in the very popular poppy seed dressing.

saffron: Saffron comes from the stamen of the crocus flower and gives a bright yellow color and wonderful flavor to rice and other dishes. Never use more saffron than is called for. Good saffron is very expensive, but the cheaper varieties are not a reasonable substitute, as they lack flavor. You'll be very disappointed. Saffron is best purchased in threads, rather than ground, because threads provide fresher flavor. Before using, saffron *must* be steeped in hot liquid to bring out its flavor.

sage: Fresh or ground sage is very pungent. It is mostly used in stuffings, sausage, and with pork.

salt: There's just no substitute for salt for adding its own flavor and for bringing out other flavors in food. Many excellent cooks, including Martha Stewart, use kosher salt because it imparts a better taste and consistency and enhances natural flavor more effectively than regular table salt. Measure for measure, kosher salt is not as strong as table salt. Others swear by sea salt's coarse crystals because it takes less salt to achieve the flavor you desire. It's often ground in a salt grinder when adding salt to cooked dishes. Rock salt is

	also used freshly ground. Seasoned salt tends to taste dehydrated and is undesirable in cooking. Experiment with all of these varieties to determine which suit you best.
turmeric:	An Indian spice made from a ground root that gives a yellow color and exotic flavor to foods.

Purchasing Herbs and Spices

Undoubtedly, your local grocery market is the most expensive source of spices and herbs. If you wish to purchase locally, first check your health food store. Many carry spices and herbs in bulk quantities, and you can measure out and purchase as much or as little as you like. *Tip:* Don't buy more than you know you will reasonably use in the next six months. It's heartbreaking to throw out expensive, albeit flat and stale, spices or herbs. Another excellent source for cheap spice is an ethnic market. For instance, curry and paprika will be less expensive in a store that caters to the Indian and Middle Eastern population. Ginger, cilantro, and soy sauce are much less expensive at an Asian market (as is rice).

At the back of this book, you will find a list of resources that includes several mail-order companies that sell herbs and spices. Call for free catalogs for each and start comparing prices. You will be amazed at the difference between your local grocery store and, say, a mail-order company. But be careful! You could easily spend all of your savings covering shipping and handling. Some mail-order companies have minimum orders, so check very carefully and take lots of time to compare.

Suzan Williams of Colorado shared some of her personal research on the subject with the readers of *Cheapskate Monthly.* Take a look at the vast difference in the costs of the most common herbs and spices:

Sample Price Comparison Chart			
One-ounce Portion	Health Food Store	Grocery Store Brand	Schilling/ McCormick
cinnamon	$.39	$.87	$2.13
garlic powder	.34	.60	2.04
parsley flakes	1.93	3.03	11.00
bay leaf	.43	13.52	30.80
basil	.28	2.96	8.62

When purchasing extracts or spices in larger quantities, consider unusual sources. *Cheapskate Monthly* reader Dolores Poepping wrote saying she needed to purchase large quantities of anise extract or anise oil. She needed to purchase by the quart or pint. (I figure that's at least an acre of anise.)

We suggested she check with local commercial bakeries. Often these companies will sell flour, sugar, extracts, parchment paper, and even yeast to customers at their cost (a fraction of what it costs you and me at the retail level). Most cities have listings in the local Yellow Pages for wholesale suppliers of everything from anise to zippers. Call. Find out what their minimum purchase is. If they can't help you, ask for a referral.

Our grocery shopping expert at *Cheapskate Monthly*, Rhonda Barfield, finally suggested Dolores contact the Olde Town Spice Shopper in St. Charles, Missouri (636) 916–3600, which at this time sells ½ ounce of oil of anise in the shop for $3.75. Call for mail order prices. I can't confirm this to be the best buy available at the time of this writing; however, it demonstrates that prices vary greatly. The careful shopper will receive great rewards for demonstrating patience and the ability to check around and compare.

Chapter 6

How to Cook
on the Cheap

The Seasonal Cook

The most important principle for conserving cash without sacrificing quality is to become a seasonal cook. Let the time of year be your guide as you plan and prepare meals. Make your salads from fresh produce that is in season when prices are lowest and quality is highest.

Meat, fish, poultry, and wild game have seasons as well. For instance, around the first part of November, turkeys appear by the carload at rock-bottom prices. If you are fortunate enough to live in an area where wild game is plentiful, hold off on those special wild game recipes until each hunting season opens and the best game is available for next to nothing (assuming someone you know is an avid hunter).

Depend on the weekly grocery ads to signal what is plentiful, thus less expensive, at any particular time of year. Because fruits and vegetables change with the seasons, your culinary repertoire should be ever-changing as well. For example, April and May offer such welcomed sights as baby greens and strawberries to be followed by the best summer has to offer in corn, tomatoes, and blueberries.

Autumn brings visions of pumpkin pies and squash delights, and why not? Harvest time has always filled our lives with fresh pumpkins, zucchinis, and apples. If you have a garden, nature itself will be calling out the best of the season. If not, let your best produce and meat market be your guide.

When deciding upon your gourmet menus, learn to think like the head chef at the finest restaurant in town. Master particular recipes that represent each of the seasons so they are at your fingertips the moment the cream of the crop is first available.

Fresh fruits and vegetables purchased at the peak of their season not only taste best, the prices will be lowest because of the rule of supply and demand. As a result of modern hothouse activities and storage techniques, we have a lot to choose from. Combine this with the shipment of produce from other parts of the world, where the seasons are reversed from ours in North America, and many fruits and vegetables become available all year around. However, during these off-peak, yet available months, the prices are much higher because of additional costs of importing. At their best, the quality of imported goods cannot match local fruits and vegetables at the peak of their seasons, especially when factoring in the cost.

Following is a chart that will help you plan your menus ahead of time.

$\diamond$ = Available $\blacklozenge$ = Peak season

	J	F	M	A	M	J	J	A	S	O	N	D
FRUITS												
Apples	$\diamond$	$\diamond$	$\diamond$	$\diamond$	$\diamond$	$\diamond$	$\diamond$	$\diamond$	$\blacklozenge$	$\blacklozenge$	$\blacklozenge$	$\blacklozenge$
Apricots					$\diamond$	$\blacklozenge$	$\blacklozenge$	$\diamond$				
Avocados	$\diamond$	$\diamond$	$\blacklozenge$	$\blacklozenge$	$\diamond$	$\diamond$	$\diamond$	$\diamond$	$\diamond$	$\diamond$	$\diamond$	$\diamond$
Bananas	$\diamond$	$\diamond$	$\blacklozenge$	$\blacklozenge$	$\blacklozenge$	$\blacklozenge$	$\diamond$	$\diamond$	$\diamond$	$\diamond$	$\diamond$	$\diamond$
Blackberries					$\diamond$	$\blacklozenge$	$\blacklozenge$	$\blacklozenge$				
Blueberries					$\diamond$	$\diamond$	$\blacklozenge$	$\blacklozenge$	$\diamond$			
Cherries					$\diamond$	$\blacklozenge$	$\blacklozenge$	$\diamond$				

	J	F	M	A	M	J	J	A	S	O	N	D
Cranberries	◇								◇	◆	◆	◇
Grapefruit	◆	◆	◆	◆	◇	◇	◇	◇	◇	◇	◆	◆
Grapes	◇	◇	◇	◇	◇	◇	◇	◇	◆	◆	◆	◇
Lemon	◇	◇	◇	◇	◇	◆	◆	◇	◇	◇	◇	◇
Limes	◇	◇	◇	◇	◇	◆	◆	◆	◇	◇	◇	◇
Melons		◇	◇	◇	◇	◇	◆	◆	◇	◇	◇	
Oranges	◆	◆	◆	◇	◇	◇	◇	◇	◇	◇	◇	◆
Peaches						◇	◆	◆	◇			
Pears	◇	◇	◇	◇	◇	◇	◇	◆	◆	◆	◇	◇
Persimmons								◇	◇	◆	◆	◇
Pineapples	◇	◇	◆	◆	◆	◆	◇	◇	◇	◇	◇	◇
Quinces	◆	◇							◇	◆	◆	◆
Raspberries					◇	◆	◇	◇	◇	◇		
Rhubarb	◇	◇	◇	◆	◆	◆	◇	◇	◇	◇	◇	◇
Strawberries	◇	◇	◇	◇	◆	◆	◇	◇	◇	◇	◇	◇
Tangerines	◆	◇	◇	◇								
Watermelons				◇	◇	◆	◆	◇	◇			
VEGETABLES												
Artichokes	◇	◇	◆	◆	◇					◇	◇	◇
Asparagus			◇	◆	◆	◆						
Beets	◇	◇	◆	◆	◇	◇	◇	◇			◇	◇
Broccoli	◆	◆	◆	◇	◇	◇	◇	◇	◇	◆	◆	◆
Brussels sprouts	◇	◇	◇					◇	◇	◆	◆	◆
Cabbage	◇	◇	◇	◇	◆	◇	◇	◇	◇	◇	◇	◇
Carrots	◆	◆	◆	◆	◆	◆	◆	◆	◆	◆	◆	◆
Cauliflower	◇	◇	◇	◇	◇	◇	◇	◇	◇	◇	◇	◇
Celery	◆	◆	◆	◆	◆	◆	◆	◆	◆	◆	◆	◆
Chard	◇	◇	◇	◇	◇	◇	◆	◆	◆	◆	◇	◇
Chicory	◇	◇	◇	◇	◇	◆	◇	◇	◇	◇	◇	◇
Collards	◆	◇	◇	◇	◇	◇	◇	◇	◇	◇	◇	◆

	J	F	M	A	M	J	J	A	S	O	N	D
Corn	◇	◇	◇	◇	◇	◆	◆	◆	◆	◇	◇	◇
Cucumbers	◇	◇	◇	◇	◇	◆	◆	◆	◆	◇	◇	◇
Dandelion greens	◇	◇	◆	◆	◆	◆	◇	◇	◇	◇	◇	◇
Eggplant	◇	◇	◇	◇	◇	◇	◆	◆	◇	◇	◇	◇
Endive	◆	◆	◆	◇	◇	◇	◇	◇	◇	◇	◆	◆
Escarole	◇	◇	◇	◇	◇	◇	◇	◇	◇	◆	◇	◇
Green beans	◇	◇	◇	◇	◆	◆	◆	◆	◇	◇	◇	◇
Green peppers	◇	◇	◇	◇	◇	◇	◆	◆	◆	◆	◇	◇
Kale	◆		◇	◇	◇	◇	◇	◇	◇	◇	◇	◆
Lettuce	◇	◇	◇	◇	◇		◇	◇	◇	◇	◇	◇
Lima beans	◇		◇	◇	◇	◇	◆	◆	◆	◆	◇	◇
Mushrooms	◇	◇	◇	◇	◇	◇	◇	◇	◇	◇	◆	◆
Mustard greens	◇	◇	◇	◇	◇	◆	◆	◇	◇	◇	◇	◇
Okra	◇	◇	◇	◇	◇	◆	◆	◇	◇	◇	◇	◇
Onions, Bermuda	◇	◇	◆	◆	◆	◆	◇	◇	◇	◇	◇	◇
Onions, green	◇	◇	◇	◇	◆	◆	◆	◆	◇	◇	◇	◇
Parsnips	◆	◆	◆	◆	◆	◆	◆	◆	◆	◆	◆	◆
Potatoes	◆	◆	◆	◆	◆	◆	◆	◆	◆	◆	◆	◆
Pumpkins									◇	◆	◇	
Radishes	◇	◇	◇	◆	◆	◆	◇	◇	◇	◇	◇	◇
Rutabagas	◆	◆	◆	◇	◇	◇	◇	◇	◇	◆	◆	◆
Spinach	◇	◇	◆	◆	◆	◆	◇	◇	◇	◇	◇	◇
Squash, summer	◇	◇	◇	◇	◆	◆	◆	◇	◇	◇	◇	◇
Squash, winter									◇	◆	◇	
Tomatoes	◇	◇	◇	◇	◇	◆	◆	◆	◆	◆	◇	◇
Turnips	◇	◇	◇	◇	◇	◇	◇	◇	◇	◆	◆	◆
Watercress	◇	◇	◇	◆	◆	◇	◇	◇	◇	◇	◇	◇
Wax beans	◇	◇	◇	◇	◆	◆	◆	◆	◇	◇	◇	◇

A Special Attitude

There's no doubt that the true food aficionado has acquired an exceptional attitude when it comes to the cost of food. While the ordinary cook settles for second best because "anything that's good costs too much," the gourmet can look at the most simple and inexpensive of foods and immediately ask, "What can I do with this to make it sensational?" The ordinary cook focuses on what is not available while the gourmet cook builds around what is available. The ordinary cook looks at the lack of money for groceries while the gourmet cook embraces the challenge of turning out delightful and creative meals with whatever amount of money might be available.

The Savvy Shopper

Experienced gourmet cooks seem to pick up a sixth sense somewhere along the line when it comes to buying food. They know where to find the bargains and how to be flexible in the face of a great unadvertised bargain. If you don't yet possess this kind of shopping savvy, focus on what these effective shoppers do and start mimicking them. Here are some of my own observations to get you going:

- Design your week's menus around the weekly grocery store sale ads. Take full advantage of the store's loss leaders (those items the store has priced below their cost in order to get you into the store).
- Make your shopping list at home when you are hungry. You will be more creative and thorough.
- Never shop hungry. You will be compelled to buy everything in sight regardless of what's on your list.
- Stick to the list. If it's not on your list, don't buy it.
- Shop with cash. If you enter the store with a checkbook or credit card, you will be more apt to buy compulsively and spend far more than you intended. While it takes a lot of courage and a bit of planning, shopping with cash is the best way to avoid expensive mistakes. If you see something that you really do need, write it down and make sure it's on your list for the next trip.

♦ Avoid convenience and specialty stores. You will not find many bargains there. However, it will be necessary to occasionally patronize these kinds of establishments, so make sure you have a list and carry cash.

♦ Shop solo. You will stick to your shopping list with much less frustration and stress if you shop alone. Kids have a way of distracting and frustrating the task at hand.

♦ Stretch fruit juices. Mix 50/50 with generic brand club soda or seltzer.

♦ Stretch concentrated fruit juice. Add more water than instructions recommend. You will be pleasantly surprised when you detect little difference, if any. Start by adding one-half of a can of water extra. Eventually work up to one full can of water over and beyond the amount recommended. This will cut your concentrated fruit juice bill by 25 percent.

♦ Make your own groceries. If you are used to purchasing a lot of preprepared foods like salad dressings, seasoning mixes, muffin and cake mixes, biscuit mixes, and hot chocolate mixes, learn how to make your own from scratch. You will save a lot of money and turn out much better-tasting foods.

♦ Learn to stretch creatively and deliciously. Oatmeal or bread crumbs stretch a pound of ground meat into a pound and a half or more; nonfat dry milk stretches a gallon of milk into two. The possibilities are endless.

♦ Buy in bulk when appropriate. Remember, it's no bargain if you end up throwing a lot of the product away because it spoiled or became stale.

♦ Keep a price book. Start keeping a notebook that lists the prices of regularly purchased items at various stores. Keep it with you so that as you see specials or ads, you'll be able to determine whether it is really a bargain or not.

♦ Do not shop when you are exhausted. You will not be as disciplined or effective.

♦ Weigh all produce even if it is priced per item or by the bag. There can be a significant difference in the weight of one bag of carrots compared to the others in the pile for example. Even with a weight printed on the bag (that number represents the minimum weight), the true weight may be quite different. Heads of lettuce priced individually can differ in weight by as much as half a pound.

Advice from Our Expert Gourmets

Ethnic food is often a great solution for the low-cost gourmet. In most ethnic recipes, meat is sparse and the food is tasty. If you read cookbooks, you soon realize only Americans think a piece of meat is a necessity.

—Julia A. Wright

Don't be wasteful. Learn to use as much of a product as possible. For example, use celery hearts (leaves and all) for soups and stews. Grow your own herbs and vegetables. Make a recipe stretch into several meals with some planning and creativity. Example: Boil a whole chicken. Use part of the broth for soup, a portion of the broth for risotto (Italian rice), and the chicken for chicken salad, casserole, or sandwiches.

—Jan Sandberg

I belong to a food co-op and get food items much cheaper as a result of that membership. I love flavored coffees but don't like to spend extra money for them, so I simply add a few shakes of cinnamon to the coffee grounds before brewing or add a drop or two of almond or vanilla extract to a fresh hot cup of coffee. I buy a huge can of tomato purée from my local grocery warehouse club. I divide it into small amounts by filling small zip-type plastic bags and placing them in the freezer until needed. After one is thawed, I add water—to make it the consistency of tomato sauce—salt, and spices for flavor. I enjoy saving money this way and also appreciate the fact that tomato purée contains no additives or preservatives.

—Paulette Hegg

Use fresh whenever possible. Invest in a basic cookbook. Turn on the Cooking Channel and use your God-given imagination! Check newspaper ads for the best prices and then create your menus around the daily specials. Buy specials in quantity if at all possible. A ratatouille can clean out the vegetable bin and cooler, and the many variations of hot soups and stews can do the same. Hors d'oeuvres are a great way to "empty" the freezer. I save the water in which the potatoes boiled to use in gravy, stews, soups, and roux; I stretch meat loaf by adding carrot peelings (diced or puréed) or grated zucchini (excellent way to get vitamins into kids without their knowledge). The meat in the cassoulet is from that delicious leftover Easter ham. Or when it's Mexican night, I serve shredded beef tacos and burritos from the beef that remained from the pot roast dinner two weeks ago. I purchase whole chickens (less expensive than cutup ones) and save the back and neck for making soup. I freeze them until I've collected enough for the amount of soup I need. Those little chicken livers can also be frozen and used for an impressive liver pâté or Rumaki.

—Mary Ann Woirhaye

Go light on the expensive foods such as meat or fish. You don't need much. Use more of the pastas, grains, fruits, and vegetables. Make your own stock from leftovers and freeze to use for flavoring in the future. Grow your own herbs and vegetables. They always taste better!

—Marilyn McCormick

Shop wisely, use fresh ingredients when possible, and pay attention to flavors more than quantity. Serve smaller quantities of the expensive things and larger portions of rolls, rice, potatoes, etc. For veal scaloppine use chicken breasts pounded and seasoned like veal; cut into thin slices the size of veal medallions. Stuff pork chops, chicken breasts, and round steak to make your meat go further and your presentation more interesting. When planning your menu, see what's on sale and work around it. Use avocados when they're 25 cents each, not $1.25 for example. Instead of mixing ingredients that stand on their own, i.e., avocados, oranges, cheeses, etc., use them as a garnish for presentation.

—Bob Kingsbury

Cheap Tips

♦ Add at least three corks to the pot to tenderize stew meat. Corks release enzymes and reduce the cooking time by as much as half. Be sure to remove corks before serving.

♦ Put cooking oil in a clean plastic spray bottle. This is much cheaper than buying oil in a spray can, and you can use the exact type of oil you want.

♦ Tired of throwing out celery that's lost its crisp and crunch? Cut off the bottom stem of a full bunch of celery and separate stalks. Fill a pan that is deep enough to cover celery with COLD water and stir in ¾ cup granulated sugar. Let celery soak for four or five hours. Drain well and refrigerate.

♦ To keep milk fresh longer, add a pinch of salt when it is first opened. It doubles the useful shelf life of milk and does not affect the taste in any way.

♦ Instead of purchasing a spaghetti measuring device from the gourmet shop, keep an empty 35mm film canister handy in your drawer of utensils. Stack uncooked spaghetti into a canister. A full canister makes spaghetti for two—no waste, no guessing.

♦ Before you put that carton of eggs into your cart, take a second to jiggle each egg to make sure it isn't stuck to the inside shell because of a crack that is not really visible. Never buy a cracked egg.

♦ Rather than spending extra dough for chicken tenderloins, pound skinless, boneless chicken breasts to about ¼-inch thickness and cut lengthwise into 2-inch by 1-inch strips.

♦ Never purchase more meat than you can properly refrigerate and reasonably use within the following periods of time: Ground beef and beef cut into small pieces, such as stew meat: use within two days of purchase. Steak: within four days. Roasts: within one week. Caution: Markets typically reduce the price of certain cuts of meat when the expiration date is imminent. Always consider these great buys as items that must be used immediately if not sooner.

♦ Meat marinades can be turned into delicious sauces. Just be sure to boil them for at least three minutes to kill any bacteria that might have been transferred from the raw meat.

♦ Tomatoes, avocados, peaches, and nectarines ripen faster when enclosed in a brown paper bag and kept at room temperature for two to three days.

Cheapstitutes

A Cheapstitute is a cheaper and better substitute for a prepared food item. Great word, huh? (I thought of it myself.) To qualify as a true Cheapstitute, the end product must be cheaper than its commercial counterpart and far superior in quality and taste. Also, all of its ingredients must be pronounceable, meaning no fillers, chemicals, or preservatives.

Following are a few of my favorite Cheapstitutes. Once you get the hang of it, I know you'll start creating your own or recognize them as you rub shoulders with other gourmets or read magazines and cookbooks.

Homemade Chicken Stock (substitute for canned chicken broth and chicken bouillon): Place some chicken necks and backs in a large pot with enough water to cover. Add a carrot, parsnip, and onion (all vegetables cut into 1- to 2-inch pieces). Bring to a boil, reduce heat, and allow to simmer covered for hours. Place in refrigerator to facilitate degreasing (once cold, scrape away and discard the hardened fat that will be sitting on the surface). Strain to remove all vegetables. Broth can be frozen for future use or used immediately.

Homemade Beef Stock (substitute for canned beef broth or bouillon): Place beef bones or one pound of ox tails in a large pot with water to cover. Add one carrot, parsnip, and onion cut into 1- or 2-inch pieces. Add black pepper to taste. Bring to a boil, reduce heat, cover, and allow to simmer many hours. Place in refrigerator to facilitate degreasing (see Chicken Stock above). Broth may be frozen or used immediately.

Master Mix (substitute for Bisquick): 5 pounds all-purpose flour, ¾ cup double-acting baking powder, 3 tablespoons salt, 2 pounds solid vegetable shortening (I swear by Crisco), 2½ cups dry milk, 2 tablespoons cream of tartar, ½ cup granulated sugar. Sift dry ingredients together. Cut in shortening until mix looks like cornmeal.

Store at room temperature in a tightly covered container, such as Tupperware. Makes 30 cups per mix. This can be used in place of Bisquick (always substituting water for milk) for biscuits, dumplings, muffins, cookies, coffee cake, pancakes, waffles, gingerbread, cornbread, and shortcake.

Maple Syrup 3 cups granulated sugar, 1½ cups water, 3 tablespoons molasses, 1 teaspoon maple extract. Bring all ingredients to a rolling boil, stirring until sugar dissolves. Turn off heat and leave pan on stove until boiling stops. Store in covered container.

Shake and Bake 1 cup bread crumbs, 2 teaspoons celery salt, 1 teaspoon garlic powder, ½ teaspoon salt, ½ cup flour, 2 teaspoons poultry seasoning, 1 teaspoon paprika, ½ teaspoon pepper, 5 teaspoons onion powder, ½ teaspoon cayenne pepper. Mix all together and store in tightly closed container. Will keep for up to four months in pantry. To use: Dip chicken pieces in mixture of ½ cup milk and one beaten egg. Pour some coating mix into a plastic bag, drop in chicken one piece at a time and shake. Bake in a greased baking dish for one hour at 375°, or until the juices run clear.

Sweetened Condensed Milk (substitute for Eagle Brand Sweetened Condensed Milk): 2 cups instant nonfat dry milk, 1½ cups sugar, ⅔ cup boiling water, 6 tablespoons butter (melted and slightly cooled). Mix dry ingredients and slowly add to boiling water. Stir in melted butter. Whip in blender or by hand until smooth. Store in refrigerator for up to one week or freeze for up to six months. Yield: 20 ounces.

Orange Julius (substitute for Orange Julius!): 2 cups orange juice, ½ cup Coffee Mate, ½ teaspoon vanilla extract, 2 tablespoons sugar, 5 large ice cubes. Place ingredients in electric blender; add ice cubes one at a time. Blend until smooth and frothy. Yield: 1–2 servings.

Hot Chocolate Mix (substitute for any hot or cold instant chocolate mix): 1 box Carnation nonfat dry milk (the size that makes 8 quarts), 1 16-ounce box confectioners sugar (any brand), 1 28-ounce jar Cremora (nondairy coffee creamer), 1 28-ounce can Hershey's Chocolate Milk Mix (*not* Hershey's Cocoa). In very large container mix these four dry ingredients well. Store in tightly covered container. To use: For hot chocolate put ⅓–½ cup mix in mug and fill with boiling water. Stir until ingredients are dissolved. For cold chocolate, put ⅓ cup mix into drinking glass and fill with cold water. Mix well until ingredients are dissolved. (Use only the brand names suggested for best results.)

Sugar-free Drink (substitute for Crystal Light): 1 cup lemon or lime juice, 5 cups cold water, 5 packets artificial sweetener. Mix all ingredients in pitcher; serve over ice.

Bread (substitute for any type of bread you need to eat within the next 75 minutes): 3 packages dry yeast, 2 eggs, 10 cups bread flour, 4 teaspoons salt, 3¾ cups warm water (115°), 6 tablespoons soft stick margarine, 6 tablespoons sugar. Dissolve yeast in warm water; add 3 teaspoons of the sugar; add remaining ingredients. Mix by hand until moist. Seal in a large 32-cup Tupperware bowl. Do not burp the bowl. When seal pops loose on its own, divide batter into four equal parts and place into greased loaf pans. Cover with a towel for thirty minutes to allow the dough to rise. Preheat oven to 350°. Bake loaves for 30 minutes. This bread freezes beautifully. For wheat bread, use 5 cups white bread flour, and 5 cups whole wheat bread flour.

Tarragon Mustard (substitute for expensive gourmet condiment): 2 cups Dijon-style mustard, 2 tablespoons minced fresh tarragon or 2 teaspoons dried, crumbled tarragon, 1 tablespoon extra-virgin olive oil, 2 teaspoons white wine vinegar, dash of cayenne pepper. In a medium bowl combine mustard, tarragon, olive oil, vinegar, and cayenne. Whisk to blend well. Refrigerate in a tightly covered container up to one month.

Spiced Honey Mustard (substitute for expensive gourmet mustard): 2 cups Dijon-style mustard, ½ cup honey, ½ teaspoon cumin, ¼ teaspoon ground allspice. In a small bowl combine mustard, honey, cumin, and allspice. Whisk to blend well. Refrigerate in a tightly covered container for up to one month.

Garlic (substitute for any fresh garlic that is not free): Every time you open a head of garlic, plant the last three or four little cloves from the center of the head and any that have begun to show green. Plant them between plants and shrubs in your yard or flower beds. Plant each clove about ½ inch deep, flat end down, pointed end up.

Garlic plants will grow to about 18 inches tall and then will start to dry out. This is the sign that it's time to pull out a fresh garlic head. It takes about five months to get your first harvest. If you're always planting, you will always have fresh garlic and lots to share for free, not three dollars a pound.

Light Coffee (substitute for any canned coffee that is half decaffeinated and half regular): Purchase equal amounts of store brand decaffeinated and regular coffee beans. Set the grinder to the very finest setting to produce European-style ground coffee. Use only a small amount of ground coffee for a pot of drip coffee. Store ground coffee in the freezer so that it retains its freshness longer.

Croutons (substitute for any pricey commercial croutons): 5 slices white or whole wheat bread, 2 tablespoons butter, 2 tablespoons olive oil, 1 teaspoon minced garlic, ½ cup freshly grated Parmesan cheese, ½ teaspoon dried crumbled oregano, ½ teaspoon dried crumbled thyme. Remove crusts from bread. Cut remaining bread in desired-size cubes. Melt butter with olive oil in a large skillet over medium heat. Add garlic and sauté about one minute. Remove pan from heat and add bread cubes, stirring until well coated with butter mixture. Cool slightly. Combine Parmesan, oregano, and thyme in heavy plastic or paper bag. Add bread cubes and toss to coat evenly with cheese mixture. Spread bread cubes in even layer on ungreased baking sheet or jelly-roll pan. Bake at 300° 35 to 40 minutes or until lightly browned and crisp, stirring occasionally. Cool, then place in freezer storage bag and freeze until needed. Makes about 2 cups of the best croutons you've ever eaten.

Garlic Salad Dressing (substitute for any commercial salad dressing): 1½ cups salad oil, 1½ teaspoons salt, ½ cup dry mustard, 4 cloves garlic (halved), ½ teaspoon dried tarragon. Mix all ingredients well and pour into a sealable jar. Let stand in sealed jar or other appropriate container overnight before serving. Store in refrigerator.

Honey Butter (substitute for any commercial spread for cornbread): Cream together honey and softened butter in any 50/50 amount. When thoroughly mixed, scoop out with a melon-baller and place honey-butter balls on a serving plate and refrigerate until time to serve.

Part Two

Creating the Pleasures of the Table

The best thing we can do is to enjoy eating,
drinking, and working. I believe these are
God's gifts to us, and no one enjoys eating
and living more than I do!
—King Solomon

$\mathcal{J}$oups, Stocks, and Sauces

No Doubt about It, the Secret's in the Sauce

*A gourmet meal has been prepared by one who has
mastered the art of cooking. Preparation, presentation,
and careful selection of the ingredients make the difference.*
—Jan Sandberg

Soups

Whether an elegant first course, the centerpiece of a meal, a sandwich's faithful luncheon companion, or a clever ploy to satiate youthful appetites, soup is a favorite resource in the thrifty gourmet's portfolio. There's nothing like a hearty soup to provide a delicious solution for what to do with the ham bone or everlasting Thanksgiving turkey.

Soup can be thick, thin, hot, cold, subtle, spicy, puréed, or creamed. It can be clear as crystal or thick and chunky. Some soups require no cooking at all; others can be prepared in thirty minutes or less, while still others require all-day simmering and taste even better when allowed to mellow in the refrigerator for a few days.

Using Leftovers in Soup

While soup is a marvelous way to utilize the remains of a previous meal or to motivate one to responsibly clear out the refrigerator bins

93

and shelves, it should never be considered tired and tasteless. In other words, soup is not a very good illusionist. An experienced cook knows what should and what should not be added to the soup or stockpot. In the beginning there's nothing like a reliable soup recipe to gain experience. You'll find some great ones at the end of this chapter.

The general rule is that soups should be cooked in a covered pot to facilitate the retention of nutrients and flavor. However, when a very thin soup needs to reduce, the pot should be only partially covered to allow for evaporation of the water and to intensify the flavors. Nothing is less satisfying than bland soup.

Seasoning Soup

Other than the bouquet garni (also called *sachet*) that is added at the beginning of classic stock and soup preparation, it is better to hold off on adding salt and pepper until the soup is nearly done. Salt added at the beginning will double or triple intensity during the reduction and simmering process, which makes it impossible to know how much to add in the beginning. Begin tasting as the soup nears the finish. Let your palate guide you in adding salt and pepper.

Storing and Freezing Soup

One of the best things about most soups: They can be prepared in advance. To keep soups from spoiling, refrigerate and reheat to boiling point every three days. Most soups freeze well, so making large batches when ingredients are plentiful and then freezing in smaller portions makes good sense.

Binding and Thickening Soup

At times soup will seem to separate or curdle, which means it needs a binder—something to hold the ingredients together. Here's the best way to bind soup: In a separate saucepan, melt 1 tablespoon of butter per 2 cups of soup. Stir an equal number tablespoons of flour into the butter, mix well, and cook over low heat for three minutes. Pour a small amount of the hot soup into the butter flour. Now add this thickened mixture to the remaining hot soup, heat, and stir until it reaches desired thickness.

Stock

Stock is the foundation ingredient for soups, sauces, and gravies. While commercial bouillon, broth, and stocks are available in canned, dried, or powdered forms (and will do in a pinch), nothing can match a good, hearty homemade stock that is free of preservatives and mystery ingredients. Stock is simply the water that has been enriched by flavorful ingredients such as meat, poultry, fish, or vegetables that have been cooked in it. Stock is full of nutrients. If you have a recipe that calls for broth, it's interchangeable with stock; the only difference between the two is that you use the meat plus the bones in making broth, and you use only the bones when making a stock. The advantage to making broth is that you now have cooked meat to use for your soup or something else.

Even though making a good stock can be time-consuming, it really is a no-brainer. There's not much you could do to spoil it provided you start with acceptable ingredients and check regularly to make sure the liquid has not boiled away.

When it comes to choosing ingredients, consider stock-making the exception to the rule since young and tender ingredients are not necessary. Actually, mature, more flavorful meat and vegetables are particularly desirable.

One of the classic foundations of a good stock is the bouquet garni (also called *sachet*). Here is how to prepare it: Place the seasonings as stated in the recipe in a square of cheesecloth. Gather up the corners and twist together. Using one end of a 12-inch piece of butcher's twine, tie the sachet closed. Tie the other end of the string to the handle of the stockpot so that it is suspended in the stock. Voila! Once you feel comfortable with this technique, you can experiment with other herbs and seasonings in stocks.

Sauces

Our gourmet panelist Jan Sandberg comes from a heritage of fine gourmet cooking. Her mother, the late Minnie Gay, created fine northern Italian fare on a daily basis, and her reputation as a gourmet extraordinare was known far and wide. One could not be in Minnie's kitchen for long without learning one valuable piece of information: The secret is in the sauce. A perfect sauce is the glorious refinement of any great meal. If you can confidently turn out an ideal sauce at the perfect moment, even the plainest of cuisine will become a masterpiece. Remember, too, that a wonderful sauce hides a multitude of cooking sins, such as tough meat, boring vegetables, or overcooked pasta.

There are five basic sauces that every serious cook needs to perfect and then know how and when to use. These are: basic béchamel sauce, basic veloute sauce, basic brown sauce (also called sauce Espagnole), basic tomato sauce, and hollandaise. Recipes for these and other basic sauces will follow at the end of the chapter.

Tips

♦ Keep a container in the freezer specifically for the collection of fresh scraps, juices, and bones that might otherwise land in the garbage. When the supply becomes sufficient, make the stock. If not needed immediately, freeze for future use.

♦ Refrigerate soups hours before serving to allow fat to solidify on the surface. Just lift off before reheating.

♦ Add a deep richness to soups by making a smoked chicken broth, using the bones and skin from a smoked chicken. Or split an onion and place cut side down in an iron skillet and place on medium heat. Let cook until the onion is burned and very black. It is very important that the onion is burnt, as it will cook with the bones in the stock for hours, creating a deep amber color and richness.

♦ Keep canned broth in the refrigerator so the fat will congeal and be easy to lift off the surface before using.

♦ Add flavor to vegetable soups by substituting a vegetable juice like V-8 for a third to half of the water in the recipe.

♦ For maximum flavor put soup bones in the soup or stew liquid before you begin heating it.

♦ Help clarify stocks by adding 2 to 3 eggshells and simmering for ten minutes. Strain off the shells before adding other ingredients.

♦ Browning meats and vegetables gives soups and stews a richer flavor.

♦ For fatty or greasy soups, if you don't have time to refrigerate, float lettuce leaves, blotting paper, or paper towel on the top. Also, make your own "grease magnet" by wrapping ice cubes in a terry cloth towel, or fill a ladle with ice cubes. The fat will cling to either.

♦ For salty soups, either increase the quantity of liquid, or if this isn't realistic, add a can of tomatoes; their blandness will use up a lot of the saltiness. Throw in a few pinches of brown sugar; the sweetness helps cover up the salty taste without sweetening the soup. Or add a thin-sliced raw potato and keep it in the broth until it becomes translucent.

♦ You can use evaporated skim milk as an ingredient when cream is called for and save more than 500 calories a cup, without sacrificing flavor. It won't whip, though.

♦ If you have problems with the gravy, consider adding any of the following (depending on the kind of gravy, that is): pungent herbs and spices; extracts such as bouillon cubes, yeast extracts, or meat extracts; bottled mixed dressings such as soy sauce, Tabasco, Worcestershire, A.1., etc.; or red currant jelly to meat gravy.

♦ Give any sauce a satiny texture by whisking in 1 or 2 tablespoons butter or whipping cream just before serving.

♦ Add color to a pale sauce or gravy by stirring in a few drops of Kitchen Bouquet (usually found in the baking/seasoning or soups/sauces section).

♦ One or two teaspoons of instant coffee powder or unsweetened cocoa powder adds both color and a rich flavor to sauces and gravies.

About Quick Canned Soup Sauces

Not only do unconcentrated canned consummes and broths perform a valuable impromptu role as strengtheners and flavoring for sauces, condensed canned soups may be used to furnish the very foundations for sauce as well. The results, of course, are not so subtle and delicate as roux-based sauces carefully constructed from fresh meat or poultry stock. But an impressive saving in time and a substantially lower caloric content go far toward offsetting loss of quality. Taste these mixtures before salting and final seasoning.

For chicken, veal, and fish, heat:
- 1 cup condensed cream of chicken soup
- 2 tablespoons butter
- 4 tablespoons chicken or vegetable sauce
  lemon zest, to taste

For creaming vegetables, heat:
- 1 cup condensed cream of celery soup
- 2 tablespoons butter
- 4 tablespoons chicken stock
- 1 tablespoon chives, chopped

Basic All-Purpose Tomato Sauce

Here is the most delicious basic tomato sauce I know. This recipe is simple to prepare, freezes well, and makes an ample supply. Every gourmet cook worth his or her sauce should always have a secret stash of tomato sauce in the freezer. Think of it as an essential in your "emergency kit." There are dozens of dishes you can prepare at a moment's notice even if your pantry is in need of restocking and guests will be arriving in thirty minutes. Learn this one well!

- 2 tablespoons olive oil
- 10 cloves garlic, chopped
- 2 onions, chopped
- 1 green bell pepper, chopped
- 1 cup fresh mushrooms, sliced

3 6 ounce cans tomato paste, plus one can water
3 12 ounce cans tomato sauce, plus one can water
1 bay leaf
3 tablespoons Italian herb seasoning

In a stockpot or large saucepan, sauté garlic, onions, green pepper, and mushrooms in olive oil. Add tomato paste, sauce, and water. Add bay leaf and Italian herb seasoning. Stir while sauce comes to a boil. Let simmer for two to three hours, uncovered, stirring occasionally. Can be used immediately or frozen in small portions for future use. Yield: 4 quarts.

Nutrient value per serving: 91 calories, 3 g protein, 2 g fat, 14 g carbohydrates, 409 mg sodium, 0 mg cholesterol.

Basic Béchamel Sauce

4 cups whole milk or cream
4 tablespoons clarified butter
4 tablespoons all-purpose flour
1 small onion, peeled
3 whole cloves
3 whole bay leaves
⅛ teaspoon ground white pepper
⅛ teaspoon freshly ground nutmeg
¼ teaspoon salt

Place the milk in a heavy saucepan and heat until scalded. Heat the clarified butter in a heavy 2-quart saucepan over medium heat. Whisk in the flour (to a paste consistency) and cook, stirring constantly for two or three minutes, until the roux bubbles and begins to color slightly. This is called a light roux.

Very gradually stir in the scalded milk. Using a hand blender, whisk continuously until smooth. Bring to a boil over medium heat. Then reduce heat and begin to simmer sauce.

Meanwhile, slice the onion in half lengthwise. Using only half the onion, pierce a whole clove through a bay leaf and then attach it to one side of the onion. Repeat with the two remaining cloves and bay leaves, attaching them around the edges of the onion. The onion will be used to flavor the sauce. Place the studded onion in the sauce and simmer uncovered for 15 to 20 minutes, stirring occasionally.

Remove and discard studded onion. Adjust the consistency of the sauce with additional hot milk, if necessary. Season to taste with salt, white pepper, and freshly ground nutmeg.

Strain the sauce though a fine strainer lined with cheesecloth. Set over a double boiler filled with warm water until ready to serve. If not using immediately, dab the top of the sauce with some butter to prevent a skin from forming. Yield: 4 cups.

Basic Beef Stock

Sachet:

2	bay leaves
10	parsley (stems only, no leaves)
4	cloves garlic
½	teaspoon whole black peppercorns
½	teaspoon dried thyme

4	pounds beef bones
	(including marrow, cut into 3–4 inch pieces)
2	onions, unpeeled
2	carrots, unpeeled
2	stalks celery
2	tablespoons tomato paste
4	quarts cold water

Preheat oven to 350°. Prepare sachet. Place bones in roasting pan and place in oven for about 30 minutes. Meanwhile, cut onions, carrots, and celery into 2-inch pieces. When bones have roasted for 30 minutes, remove pan from oven and add onions, carrots, and celery. Return to oven and roast for about 20 minutes longer. Brush the bones with tomato paste, coating all sides, and return pan to oven for 15 to 20 minutes longer. Transfer bones and vegetables to a heavy, 8-quart stockpot. Drain off fat from roasting pan. Using a little water to loosen the brown particles on the bottom of the roasting pan, deglaze the pan and transfer that liquid to the stockpot. Cover bones and vegetables with remaining cold water. Drop in the pre-made sachet. Bring to a boil, skimming off any impurities from the surface. Reduce heat and simmer, uncovered, for 4 to 6 hours, skimming off any impurities from the surface as needed. Untie sachet from the pot. Pour stock and sachet into a strainer lined with several layers of dampened cheesecloth. Use a ladle or large spoon to gently press any remaining vegetables through strainer. Discard bones and sachet. Allow the strained stock to cool completely. Cover and store in the refrigerator in an airtight container for up to 1 week. Stock may also be frozen for up to 3 months. Yield: 4 quarts.

Basic Brown Sauce (Sauce Espagnole)

Sachet:
½ bay leaf
2 parsley (stems only, no leaves)
⅛ teaspoon dried thyme
1 clove garlic

1 small onion, peeled
1 carrot, peeled
1 stalk celery
½ cup flour
½ cup clarified butter
2 tablespoons additional clarified butter
6 cups basic beef stock, brought to room temperature
2 ounces tomato puree
⅛ teaspoon salt
⅛ teaspoon ground white pepper

Make sachet. Cut the onion, carrot, and celery into ½-inch pieces. Set aside. Heat the ½ cup of clarified butter in small saucepan until hot. Whisk in the flour (to a paste consistency) and cook over medium heat, stirring constantly for 8–10 minutes until the roux bubbles, turns light brown in color, and has a nutty aroma (a dark roux). Set aside.

Place the remaining 2 tablespoons of clarified butter in a heavy 4-quart stockpot over medium heat. Add the onion, carrot, and celery. Sauté the vegetables, stirring often, for about 6–8 minutes or until well browned. Add the cooked roux to the vegetables, stirring to combine. Gradually, pour in the brown stock and then the tomato purée. Tie the sachet to one handle of the stockpot and let it dangle in the liquid. Bring to a boil, skimming off any impurities from the surface, as needed. Reduce heat and simmer uncovered for about 2 hours, skimming the surface occasionally until the sauce is reduced to about 1 quart.

Untie sachet. Pour sauce and sachet into a fine strainer lined with dampened cheesecloth. Use a ladle or spoon to gently press any remaining vegetables through the strainer. Discard the sachet. Season to taste with salt and white pepper, if desired. Set over a double boiler filled with warm water until ready to serve. Or cool completely, then cover and store in the refrigerator in an airtight container for up to one week. Sauce may also be frozen for up to 3 months. Yield: 1 quart.

Basic Chicken Stock

Sachet:

2	bay leaves
10	parsley (stems only, no leaves)
½	teaspoon dried thyme
12 to 14	whole black peppercorns

3	pounds chicken bones (wings, back, and necks)
2	large onions, peeled
2	large carrots, peeled
2	stalks celery
4	quarts cold water

Prepare sachet and tie to stockpot handle. Rinse bones well under cold running water. Cut the onions, carrots, and celery into large (¾-inch) pieces. Place bones in a heavy, 6-quart stockpot. Add onions, carrots, and celery and pour in the cold water. There should be enough to completely cover the bones. Drop in the sachet. Bring to a boil, skimming off any impurities from the surface. Reduce heat and simmer uncovered for 2 to 3 hours, skimming off any impurities from the surface as needed. Untie the sachet. Pour stock (and sachet) into a strainer lined with several layers of dampened cheesecloth. Cover and store in the refrigerator in an airtight container for up to 1 week. Stock may be frozen for up to 3 months. Yield: 4 quarts.

Basic Fish Stock

Sachet:

2	bay leaves
8	parsley (stems only, no leaves)
½	teaspoon dried thyme
14 to 18	whole black peppercorns
2	pounds fish bones, tails, and heads (gills removed)
1	tablespoon butter
1	small onion, peeled
1	stalk celery
8	cups cold water

Prepare sachet and tie to handle of stockpot. Clean fish bones thoroughly under running water. Dice the onion and celery. Melt butter in a heavy, 6-quart stockpot. When hot, add onion and celery. Sauté the vegetables over medium heat, stirring occasionally, for 3 to 5 minutes or until onion is translucent. Place bones on top of vegetables and cover with a piece of parchment paper. Reduce heat to low and cook on low for about 5 minutes. Remove and discard parchment paper. Bring to a simmer. Add the water which should be enough to cover the bones completely. Drop in the sachet. Simmer uncovered for 25 to 30 minutes, skimming off any impurities from the surface. Untie the sachet. Pour stock and sachet into a strainer lined with several layers of dampened cheesecloth. Use a ladle or large spoon to gently press any remaining vegetables through the strainer. Discard bones and sachet. Allow the strained stock to cool completely. Cover and store in the refrigerator in an airtight container for up to 1 week. Stock may be frozen for up to 3 months. Yield: 6 cups.

Basic Hollandaise

3   egg yolks
3   tablespoons water
¼   teaspoon fresh lemon juice, strained
⅛   teaspoon cayenne pepper
⅛   teaspoon salt
¾   cup clarified butter (keep warm)

In the top of a double boiler, whisk together egg yolks, water, lemon juice, cayenne, and salt. Cook over low heat, whisking vigorously, until mixture is creamy and reaches the ribbon stage.

Remove mixture from heat but continue whisking. Add the clarified butter, very slowly at first, by dropping in no more than 1 teaspoonful at a time. After a total of 2 to 3 tablespoons of butter have been whisked in and absorbed, add the remaining butter in a slow, very thin stream. Continue whisking vigorously. Taste and adjust seasoning as desired.

Sauce may be kept warm for 15 minutes over a double boiler on very low heat. The water should not exceed 150°. If the sauce separates, place one egg yolk in a clean pan over a double boiler filled with 150° water. Whisk to a light froth. Remove from heat and slowly add the separated sauce to the cooked egg yolk, whisking vigorously until completely combined. Yield: 1 cup.

Basic Mayonnaise

 4 egg yolks
1½ teaspoons Dijon mustard
    salt, to taste
 1 tablespoon lemon juice
1½ cups olive oil

Place the egg yolks and mustard in the bowl of a food processor fitted with a metal blade. Process with on/off bursts for about 30 seconds or until blended. Add the lemon juice and process for about 15 seconds longer. This next step is very critical, and it must be done slowly: with the machine running on low speed, add just a few drops of oil to begin with. Continue adding oil a few drops at a time in a slow steady stream.

As the mixture begins to thicken slightly, begin to add the oil a little faster. You should still be adding the oil slowly in a steady stream. Continue adding oil until all has been incorporated and the mixture has emulsified.

Season to taste with salt as needed. If the mayonnaise appears too stiff, add a few drops of water, stirring to combine. Transfer to an airtight container and store in the refrigerator for up to 24 hours.

Note: If you add the oil too fast or the mayonnaise separates, place an egg yolk in a small bowl and whisk in the separated mayonnaise, just a little at a time. Continue to whisk vigorously, adding small amounts of mayonnaise each time until mixture has thickened. Yield: 2 cups.

Basic Vegetable Stock

Sachet:
- 1   bay leaf
- 1   teaspoon dried oregano leaves
- 4   sprigs parsley

- 2   leeks, cleaned
- 1   yellow onion, peeled
- 2   stalks celery
- 2   small carrots
- 1   turnip, peeled
- 1   parsnip, peeled
- 1   potato, unpeeled
- ½   pound mushrooms
- 2   tablespoons vegetable oil
- 9   cloves garlic, crushed
- 2   tablespoons miso (fermented soybean paste)
- ½   teaspoon ground white pepper
- 10 cups water

Prepare sachet and suspend from handle of the stockpot. Cut leeks, onion, and celery into ½-inch pieces. Slice carrots, turnip, and parsnip into ½-inch rounds. Cut the potato into quarters and cut the mushrooms in half. Heat the oil in a heavy, 6-quart stockpot. When the oil is hot, add the leeks, onions, and carrots. Cook over medium heat, stirring occasionally, for about 5 minutes. Add the celery, parsnip, turnip, potato, and mushrooms. Add the garlic, miso, ground white pepper and cold water, stirring to combine. Drop in the sachet so that it is suspended in the mixture. Bring to a boil, skimming off any impurities from the surface. Reduce heat and simmer uncovered for 30 to 35 minutes. Continue to skim off any impurities as needed. Untie the sachet. Pour stock and sachet into a strainer lined with several layers of dampened cheesecloth. Use a ladle or large spoon to gently press any remaining vegetables through the strainer. Discard the sachet. Allow the strained stock to cool completely. Cover and store in the refrigerator in an airtight container for up to one week. Stock may be frozen for up to 3 months. Yield: 2 quarts.

Basic Veloute Sauce

2 cups basic chicken stock or basic fish stock
3 tablespoons butter
3 tablespoons all-purpose flour
⅛ teaspoon salt
⅛ teaspoon ground white pepper

Place the stock in a small saucepan and bring to a boil. Turn off the heat and set aside. Melt the butter in a heavy, 2-quart saucepan over low heat. Whisk in the flour (to a paste consistency) and cook over medium heat, stirring constantly, for 2 to 3 minutes until the roux bubbles and begins to color slightly.

Remove the roux from the heat and allow to cool slightly. Gradually pour in the hot stock, whisking continuously until smooth. Return pan to heat and bring to a boil over medium heat, whisking constantly.

Reduce heat and simmer uncovered for about 5 minutes. Season to taste with salt and white pepper, if desired. Set over a double boiler filled with warm water until ready to serve. If not using immediately, dab the top of the sauce with some butter to prevent a skin from forming. Yield: 2 cups.

French Tomato Sauce

3   tablespoons olive oil
4   ounces bacon, diced
1   cup chopped carrots
1   cup chopped onions
¼   cup all-purpose flour
6½ pounds tomatoes, skinned, seeded, and diced
1   tablespoon chopped garlic
4   cups basic vegetable stock or basic chicken stock
1½ tablespoons sugar
    salt and pepper to taste

In a large stockpot, heat oil and add the bacon. Cook until slightly crispy. Add the carrots and onions, cover, and cook slowly for 20 minutes. Dust the flour over the vegetables and cook until the flour turns golden. Add the tomatoes, garlic, and stock. Bring to a boil, reduce heat, and simmer for 2 hours. Add the sugar and season with salt and pepper. Carefully purée with a hand mixer and strain through a fine sieve. Yield: 1½ quarts.

Fresh Tomato Salsa
Contributed by Margaret Gamble

5   tomatoes, diced
⅓   cup tomato sauce
¼   cup red onions, finely chopped
2   cloves garlic, minced
1   jalapeño, seeded and minced
2   tablespoons fresh parsley, chopped
1   teaspoon dried oregano
1   teaspoon salt
2   tablespoons lime juice

Combine all ingredients, stirring gently; cover and chill. Serve with tortilla chips. Yield: 2 cups.

Fresh Tomato Soup

1   small onion, finely chopped
2   tablespoons butter
1½ cups water
2   tomatoes, cut into chunks
2   tablespoons fresh parsley, finely chopped
2   cups half-and-half
1   cup milk
    salt and pepper, to taste
2   tablespoons butter
1   tablespoon fresh dill weed, chopped
4   tablespoons sour cream

In medium skillet, sauté chopped onion in butter until onions are translucent. Add water, tomato chunks, and parsley. Simmer for 10 minutes. Purée in blender. Heat half-and-half and milk in skillet; add tomato mixture. Season with salt and pepper. Add butter and dill weed. Garnish each serving with dollop of sour cream and sprig of parsley.

Nutrient value per serving: 361 calories, 7 g protein, 31 g fat, 14 g carbohydrates, 500 mg sodium, 90 mg cholesterol.

Harvest Stew in a Pumpkin Shell
10 Servings

      2 pounds stew meat, cut into 1-inch cubes
      ¼ cup flour
     1½ teaspoons salt
      ½ teaspoon pepper
      2 cups beef broth
      1 teaspoon Worcestershire sauce
      1 clove garlic
      1 bay leaf
      1 teaspoon paprika
      4 carrots, sliced
      3 potatoes, diced
      2 onions, chopped
      1 celery stalk, chopped
      2 teaspoons Kitchen Bouquet, optional*
      ½ cup quick-cooking tapioca
      1 10 ounce package frozen peas
      1 medium pumpkin
         butter, melted
         *look for this liquid in spice section of store

Place meat in slow cooker or large casserole. Mix flour, salt, and pepper and pour over meat; stir to coat meat. Add remaining ingredients (except for pumpkin and melted butter) and stir to mix well. Cover and cook on low setting for 10 hours (high for four hours) if using a slow cooker, or bake at 250° for six hours. Prior to end of cooking time, cut top off pumpkin. Scoop out seeds and stringy membrane. Brush inside of pumpkin with butter and sprinkle lightly with salt and pepper. After end of cooking time, stir stew and spoon into pumpkin shell. Place shell in a shallow pan and bake at 325° for one hour or until pumpkin meat is tender. Place pumpkin in large bowl and ladle out stew, scooping out some of the pumpkin with each serving.

Nutrient value per serving: 393 calories, 23 g protein, 18 g fat, 35 g carbohydrates, 611 mg sodium, 71 mg cholesterol.

Lemon-Butter Sauce for Fish

This delicious sauce goes well over salmon, trout, sole, and turbot.

½ lemon, zest only
2 tablespoons fresh lemon juice
¼ cup chicken stock or fish stock
  salt and freshly ground white pepper
10 tablespoons unsalted butter, cut into ¼-inch slices
  minced fresh green herbs like parsley, dill, and/or chives
  (optional)

Bring the lemon zest, lemon juice, and the stock or broth to a boil in a 6-cup saucepan with salt and grinds of pepper. Boil slowly for several minutes until reduced to a syrup. Start whisking in the butter piece by piece, adding a new piece as each previous one is almost absorbed. Remove from heat as soon as the last piece of butter is incorporated, and whisk in herbs if being used. Serve immediately. Yield: ¾ cup.

Potato Cheese Soup

Contributed by Lori Hubert
6 Servings

6 potatoes, medium-sized, peeled, and diced
1 16 ounce package American cheese, such as Velveeta
6 slices bacon
1 onion, medium-sized, chopped
1 carrot, sliced and diced
1 teaspoon dried basil
1 teaspoon salt
1 teaspoon pepper
1 teaspoon dried parsley
1 teaspoon dried thyme

Place bite-sized pieces of potato in large saucepan with enough water to cover and bring to a boil. Cut up carrots and add to potatoes. Cook bacon until crisp. Sauté onion in bacon grease. When potato and water begin to thicken and vegetables are soft, add herbs and spices. Crumble bacon and add along with the onion. Just before serving, cut up cheese and stir in until melted. Soup should be very thick. Enjoy!

Nutrient value per serving: 409 calories, 15 g protein, 14 g fat, 56 g carbohydrates, 1,142 mg sodium, 31 mg cholesterol.

Quick and Healthy Lentil Soup
Contributed by Toni Lopopolo
4 Servings

     3 carrots
3 to 4 stalks celery
     1 bunch parsley
     1 large yellow onion
     4 cloves garlic, peeled
     2 cups lentils
       salt and pepper
       olive oil
       green onion tops, finely chopped
       parmesan cheese
       spinach leaves

Chop carrots, celery stalks, yellow onion, parsley, and garlic. Pour into saucepan along with dry lentils. Cover with water, salt to taste, and simmer for 30 minutes.

Line soup bowls with fresh clean spinach leaves. Ladle soup over leaves. The heat of soup will cook spinach perfectly. Garnish with a bit of olive oil, fresh green chopped onion, and Parmesan cheese. (Spinach treatment is optional, but very classy!)

Simply Elegant Black Bean Soup
Contributed by Nancy Guth
8 Servings

2 16 ounce cans black beans (Sun Vista brand, if available)
1 16 ounce can Mexican-style stewed tomatoes (S&W brand,
     if available)
1 12 ounce can shoepeg corn

Garnish:
½ cup sour cream
    cilantro

Open the cans. Do not drain. Dump everything into large pot and heat thoroughly.

Serve with a dollop of sour cream and chopped cilantro. Serve with Mexican cornbread. Shhhhhh. No one will even dream you haven't slaved over a hot stove all afternoon!

Split Pea Soup
6 Servings

Stock:
2 quarts bones and scraps from a cooked ham
3 quarts water or chicken stock
1 cup carrots, peeled and chopped
1 cup onions, peeled and chopped
1 stalk celery, with leaves, washed and chopped

Herb Bouquet (tie all inside a piece of cheesecloth):
3 bay leaves
1 teaspoon thyme
5 cloves
    salt

Soup:
3 tablespoons butter

⅔ cup celery, diced
⅔ cup onions, diced
½ cup carrots, diced
½ cup rutabagas, diced
3 tablespoons flour
2 quarts ham stock
1½ cups split peas
   salt and freshly ground pepper

Garnish:
1½ cups croutons
½ cup ham, diced

Stock: Chop up the ham bones and put them in a large stockpot with water to cover by 2 inches. Add the ham scraps, chopped vegetables, and herb bouquet. Simmer 3 to 4 hours partially covered to allow for air circulation; salt lightly after an hour or so, and skim impurities off of surface. Strain and degrease.

In a large saucepan, melt butter over high heat and sauté the vegetables, stirring frequently for about five minutes. Blend in the flour; cook, stirring, for three minutes. Remove from heat and let cool briefly; blend in the ham stock that has been heated, then the split peas. Bring to a simmer, stirring constantly. Cover loosely and simmer about 45 minutes or until the peas are tender. Salt and pepper to taste after ½ hour of simmering.

Purée the soup in a food processor.

Serving: Ladle the hot soup into bowls and garnish with croutons and ham dices that have been sautéed in butter.

Nutrient value per serving: 852 calories, 77 g protein, 33 g fat, 61 g carbohydrates, 4,407 mg sodium, 170 mg cholesterol.

Tartar Sauce for Fish

1½ cups mayonnaise (preferably made from scratch)
3 tablespoons capers, minced
1 small sour dill pickle, minced
2 eggs, hard-boiled
3 tablespoons fresh herbs such as parsley, tarragon, and
   chives, minced
   salt, freshly ground white pepper, lemon juice, Dijon-style
   mustard

Place mayonnaise in a small mixing bowl. Drain juices from pickle
and capers and stir into mayonnaise. Halve the eggs and take out
yolks. Force yolks through a sieve into the bowl. Chop and add the
egg whites. Add the herbs, blend all together, and season to taste.

Tortilla Soup
Contributed by Nancy Guth
6 Servings

2 cups water
14½ ounces beef broth
14½ ounces chicken broth
14½ ounces tomatoes, chopped
½ cup onions, chopped
¼ cup green bell peppers, chopped
2 boneless chicken breasts, skinned
8¾ ounces whole kernel corn, drained
1 teaspoon chili powder
½ teaspoon ground cumin
⅛ teaspoon black pepper
3 cups coarsely ground tortilla chips
4 ounces Monterey Jack cheese, shredded
1 avocado, peeled, seeded, and cubed
   cilantro (optional)
   lime wedges (optional)

In a large saucepan, combine water, beef and chicken broth, undrained tomatoes, onion, and green pepper. Bring to a boil. Cut chicken into 1-inch cubes and add to saucepan. Reduce heat, cover, and simmer for 10 minutes. Add corn, chili powder, cumin, and black pepper. Simmer, covered, for 10 more minutes. Place crushed tortilla chips into bowl and ladle soup over chips. Sprinkle with cheese, avocado, and cilantro. Serve with lime wedges.

Nutrient value per serving: 465 calories, 28 g protein, 24 g fat, 35 g carbohydrates, 987 mg sodium, 70 mg cholesterol.

Chapter 8

$\mathscr{B}$reads

THE GOURMET COOK IS WELL-BREAD

Don't murder the yeast.
—Julia Child

Bread, the staff of life, pure comfort—heaven! I really like bread. In fact, I have no doubt I could survive for a very long time on nothing more than good quality, preferably homemade, bread.

While I'm sure there is an official list declaring the categories of bread, to me there are only two: quick breads and yeast breads.

Quick Breads

Muffins, biscuits, and fruit and vegetable loaves are typical of quick breads. The leavening agent in quick breads is baking powder, baking soda, eggs, or a combination thereof. There is not a requirement for quick breads to rise prior to baking and thus their designation as "quick."

When making quick breads, it is very important to follow the directions carefully, mixing all of the dry ingredients and adding the liquid only at the very last minute before it goes into a preheated oven. Why? Because the leavening agent (baking soda or baking powder) starts working immediately upon being introduced to liquid. It starts emitting gases that will make the dough rise but will run out of gas quickly if left on the counter or otherwise delayed.

117

Yeast Breads

Making yeast bread is for those who love to spend a lot of time in the kitchen getting their hands messy. I get a great sense of satisfaction from the feel of a good yeast dough, its smell and personality. Perhaps because the process is generally long and often tedious, making bread for me is a kind of relationship. The art of making bread is not something you will learn overnight. It's like any art form—there's always something new to learn.

Yeast

Always keep in mind that yeast is a living thing; at least it's supposed to be at the moment you begin making your bread. There's nothing more frustrating than spending hours working on the perfect dough only to learn hours later that the yeast is dead. It is important to start with a fresh, quality yeast. I pay a little bit more but purchase French baking yeast in my grocery store. It comes in bulk, and I store it in the freezer tightly wrapped in two sealable bags.

Active dry yeast comes in ¼-ounce envelopes; it can also be purchased in jars or in bulk at natural food stores. Active dry yeast comes in two varieties—regular and quick-rising. Both versions can be used interchangeably, measure for measure.

Compressed, fresh yeast is sold in .6- ounce and 2-ounce "cakes." This form of yeast is very moist and goes bad quickly if not handled properly. Be sure to pay attention to the printed expiration date. Before using compressed yeast, bring it to room temperature.

Proofing Yeast

Any master baker starts with this important step: making the yeast defend itself and prove that it is indeed alive and up to the task at hand. To proof yeast, dissolve a package or tablespoon of it in 3 tablespoons of warm water (between 105° and 110°). Whisk in ¼ teaspoon of sugar to "feed" it. Look at it in about five minutes. If it has begun to get foamy, it is alive and ready to go to work. A good yeast bread recipe will give proving instructions.

Rising

Dough must be placed in a perfectly climate-controlled area for perfect rising. If the area is more than 80°, it will rise too quickly and the flavor will be decreased. If the area is drafty and less than 70° it will not rise properly. I've found the perfect environment in my oven. I turn the oven on to 350° for exactly 1½ minutes, turn it off, set the dough inside the oven and close the door. You may need to experiment with your particular area and oven to find that perfect rising environment.

Making Your Own Baker's Oven

It's acceptable to bake bread on baking sheets or in bread pans; however, you'll never achieve the size of loaf and quality of crust with pans. Here's how to turn your oven into a real baker's oven:

Purchase terra-cotta quarry tiles at your local home improvement center. Make sure they are not sealed or glazed. I have two 12-inch square tiles and several 4-inch squares that have been cut. I place a rack at the very lowest point in the oven and my tiles cover it completely, almost like puzzle pieces. I bake the bread right on the tiles, thus replicating an authentic French baking oven. It's important, too, that when baking bread you have a source of steam. I throw about ¼–½ cup of water onto the floor of the oven, which creates just the right amount of steam to make the bread very crusty.

Learn from a Master

If after trying a few recipes that follow, you get the bug to really master the bread-baking craft, I recommend you get Julia Child's excellent book *The Way to Cook*. In my opinion she's the best. Her tome is filled with detailed photos and explanations that go through each step in detail.

Tips

- ♦ Add nutrition to any bread with the Cornell Enrichment Formula. Before measuring flour into the measuring cup, add 1 tablespoon each soy flour and nonfat milk powder and 1 teaspoon wheat germ. Spoon in flour and level off. Repeat for each cup of flour used in the recipe.

- ♦ One beaten large egg has a leavening power equal to ½ teaspoon baking powder.

- ♦ For extra leavening in loaves that contain a lot of heavy ingredients, substitute 1 beaten large egg for ¼ cup of the liquid called for in the recipe.

- ♦ Bread made without fat—like French bread—has a shorter shelf life than those with fat because fat holds moisture in baked goods.

- ♦ Too much baking powder or baking soda gives quick bread a crumbly, dry texture and bitter undertaste. It can also make the batter overrise, causing the bread to fall.

- ♦ Too little baking powder or baking soda produces a bread with a heavy, gummy texture. For a delicious, triflelike dessert, cut overly dry sweet quick bread into 1-inch chunks, drizzle with fruit juice, and layer with fresh berries or other fruit and pudding or whipped cream. Cover and refrigerate for 4 hours before serving.

Dutch Baby
6 Servings

Also referred to as a German baby, baked pancake, or oven pancake, this sweet pancake is said to have originated in a small family restaurant in Seattle. The egg batter is similar to Yorkshire pudding. It is baked in the oven in a shallow pan until puffy and golden and is usually served with a dusting of powdered sugar and fresh fruit.

    1   cup all-purpose flour
    1   tablespoon sugar
  1¼ cups whole milk

    2   eggs
    ¼   teaspoon salt
    1   tablespoon unsalted butter
        powdered sugar
        slices of fruit or berries

Preheat oven to 375°. Melt butter in pan. In large bowl combine flour, sugar, milk, eggs, and salt. Stir until combined. Pour batter into pan and bake for 30 minutes until edges have risen and are golden brown and center is set. Remove from oven and dust with powdered sugar. Serve with fresh fruit.

Nutrient value per serving: 159 calories, 6 g protein, 5 g fat, 22 g carbohydrates, 144 mg sodium, 83 mg cholesterol.

Flour Tortilla Baskets
1 Serving

        10-inch flour tortillas
        oil

Brush both sides of each flour tortilla with oil. Preheat oven to 375°. Drape tortillas over ovenproof bowls and place on cookie sheets. Bake until lightly brown, about 10 minutes. Remove from oven and allow to cool while still draped over bowls. Use these for taco and other salads.

Dessert Tortilla Baskets:

Trim small flour tortillas with ravioli cutter and brush both sides with oil. Press into large muffin cups or small fluted molds. Sprinkle with sugar and/or cinnamon (1 tablespoon cinnamon to ¼ cup sugar). Bake as above.

Focaccia
8 Servings

This Italian flat onion bread is a delicious accompaniment to any meal of pasta and salad.

1   package quick-rise active dry yeast
1   teaspoon salt
2   cups all-purpose flour
    olive oil
1   cup whole wheat flour
1   tablespoon cornmeal
1   red onion, sliced
2   tablespoons Parmesan cheese, grated
1   tablespoon fresh rosemary, OR 1 teaspoon dried rosemary
¼   teaspoon cracked black pepper
    coarse salt
¼   cup thinly sliced dried tomatoes in oil (optional)

About two hours before serving or earlier in the day:

In a large bowl combine yeast, salt, and 1 cup all-purpose flour. In a 1-quart saucepan over medium heat, heat 2 tablespoons olive oil and 1 cup water until very warm (125° to 130°). With mixer at low speed, beat liquid into dry ingredients just until blended. Increase speed to medium; beat 2 minutes. Add ½ cup all-purpose flour; beat 2 minutes. Stir in whole wheat flour.

Knead dough about 8 minutes, working in about ½ cup of remaining flour. Cover and let rest 15 minutes.

Grease 13 x 9-inch pan; sprinkle with cornmeal. Pat dough into pan, pushing dough well into corners. Cover; let rise in warm place until doubled, about 30 minutes.

In 2-quart saucepan over medium heat, add 1 tablespoon olive oil and cook sliced onion until tender.

Preheat oven to 400°. With your finger, make deep indentations over entire surface of dough; drizzle with 1 tablespoon olive oil; top with onion, Parmesan, rosemary, tomatoes, pepper, and coarse salt.

Bake bread 20 to 25 minutes until golden. Cut into squares to serve.

Nutrient value per serving: 208 calories, 7 g protein, 3 g fat, 39 g carbohydrates, 468 mg sodium, 1 mg cholesterol.

Herbed Garlic Pita Toasts
12 Servings

¾ cup butter, melted
1 tablespoon fresh dill weed, OR 1 teaspoon dried dill weed
1 tablespoon fresh parsley, minced
1 clove garlic, minced
   juice of ½ lemon
6 pita breads, separated horizontally and each half cut
   into 2 pieces

To the melted butter add dill, parsley, garlic, and lemon juice. Brush mixture onto inside of each pita piece. Arrange buttered side up in one layer on a baking sheet. Bake in a 450° preheated oven for 5 minutes or until lightly browned and crisp.

Nutrient value per serving: 156 calories, 2 g protein, 12 g fat, 10 g carbohydrates, 225 mg sodium, 31 mg cholesterol.

Lemon Muffins
6 Servings

1¾ cups flour
½ cup plus 3 tablespoons sugar
1 tablespoon baking powder
½ teaspoon salt
1 egg
⅔ cup milk
1 tablespoon lemon zest, minced
1 tablespoon lemon juice
⅓ cup oil

Preheat oven to 400°. Combine flour, ½ cup sugar, baking powder, and salt in medium-sized mixing bowl. Beat egg lightly in small bowl. Stir in milk, 2½ teaspoons lemon zest, lemon juice, and oil. Add liquid to flour mixture, stirring just until moistened. Fill 6 large or 12 small greased muffin cups ⅔ full. Combine remaining 3 tablespoons sugar and ½ teaspoon lemon zest. Sprinkle over tops of muffins. Bake for 20 minutes. After baking, muffins should have rounded tops and cauliflower-like surfaces.

Note: Raw or decorator sugar may be substituted for granulated sugar in topping.

Nutrient value per serving: 271 calories, 6 g protein, 14 g fat, 30 g carbohydrates, 393 mg sodium, 39 mg cholesterol.

Master Mix
10 Dozen Biscuits

5 pounds all-purpose flour
2½ cups instant low-fat dry milk
½ cup sugar
¾ cup double-acting baking powder
2 tablespoons cream of tartar
3 tablespoons salt
2 pounds solid vegetable shortening

Sift dry ingredients together. Cut in shortening until mix looks like cornmeal. Store at room temperature in Tupperware or similar container(s). Makes 30 cups and can be used in place of Bisquick, substituting water for milk.

One dozen biscuits: 3 cups master mix, ¾ cup water. Blend and knead a few strokes. Roll out and cut out. Bake 10 minutes at 450°.

Nutrient value per serving: 299 calories, 6g protein, 16 g fat, 34 g carbohydrates, 609 mg sodium, 0 mg cholesterol.

Mexican Cornbread
Contributed by Nancy Guth
6 Servings

1   stick butter
¼   cup sugar
2   eggs
1   8 ounce can creamed corn
1   6 ounce can green chilies, diced
¼   cup Jack cheese, shredded
¼   cup cheddar cheese, shredded
½   cup flour
½   cup yellow cornmeal
2   teaspoons baking powder

With electric mixer, cream together butter and sugar. Add eggs, stir in chilies, corn, and cheeses. Sift together the dry ingredients and add to corn mixture. Pour into greased 8 x 8-inch baking dish. Bake at 300° for one hour. (Optional: prepare in muffin tin; bake for 50 minutes at 325° or until done when tested by inserting toothpick into center and it comes out clean.)

Nutrient value per serving: 204 calories, 7 g protein, 4 g fat, 28 g carbohydrates, 214 mg sodium, 85 mg cholesterol.

Mother's Herb Bread
10 Servings

1   cup butter, softened
1   teaspoon garlic powder
1   teaspoon beau monde seasoning
1   teaspoon celery flakes
1   teaspoon sage
½   teaspoon summer savory
½   teaspoon rosemary
½   teaspoon thyme
½   teaspoon basil
½   teaspoon oregano
½   teaspoon chervil
3   tablespoons parsley, minced
1   loaf sourdough bread, sliced

Combine butter, garlic powder, beau monde, celery flakes, sage, summer savory, rosemary, thyme, basil, oregano, chervil, and parsley. Stir well to blend.

Spread between slices of bread, brushing any remaining on top. Wrap securely in foil and bake at 350° for 30 minutes.

Nutrient value per serving: 269 calories, 5 g protein, 20 g fat, 18 g carbohydrates, 390 mg sodium, 50 mg cholesterol.

Orange-Raisin Muffins
16 Servings

1   cup sugar
½   cup unsalted butter
2   eggs
1   teaspoon baking soda
1   cup buttermilk
2   cups flour
½   teaspoon salt
1   cup raisins
    orange peel, from one orange

orange juice, from one orange
½ cup sugar

Preheat oven to 400°. Butter medium-sized muffin tins. With an electric mixer cream the sugar and butter until smooth. Add the eggs and beat until fluffy. Add the baking soda to the buttermilk. Sift the flour and salt together, and add to the sugar-butter-egg mixture alternately with the buttermilk. Stir until mixed. In a food grinder or processor, grind the raisins and orange peel (make sure you include only the orange peel, not the white layer next to the fruit). Add to the batter and combine. Spoon the batter into the prepared muffin tins and bake until golden brown and firm to the touch, about 12 minutes. Remove the tins to a baking rack and set close together. Brush the tops of the muffins with the orange juice and sprinkle with the remaining ½ cup sugar while still warm. Cool before serving.

Nutrient value per serving: 255 calories, 3 g protein, 7 g fat, 45 g carbohydrates, 150 mg sodium, 43 mg cholesterol.

Spiced Brioche
12 Servings

This is a basic sweet yeast dough that can be used to make cinnamon rolls, sweet bread, and coffee cake.

To prove yeast:
1 package active dry yeast
3 tablespoons water, lukewarm, not less than 105° and
    not more than 110°
2 teaspoons sugar

To make the dough:
3½ cups all-purpose flour
1½ teaspoons salt
⅓ cup sugar
½ to 1 teaspoon cinnamon
6 ounces unsalted butter, chilled and cut into pieces
    (1½ sticks)

    4 large eggs
    ⅓ cup milk, you may need a little more

Blend the perfectly warmed water, yeast, and sugar in a small bowl
or measuring cup. Stir gently and allow to sit for 5 minutes. If it
begins to foam, continue. If not, start proving process again with
fresh yeast.

Pour the flour, salt, sugar, and cinnamon into the bowl of your
food processor. Drop the chilled butter into the flour mixture. Pulse
by quick bursts to break the butter. Continue on and off until the
flour looks like rough pebbles.

Whisk the eggs and ⅓ cup of milk with the yeast mixture what has
been proving. Turn on the machine and slowly pour this liquid
almost a drop at a time into the pouring tube of the food processor.
The dough will start forming a ball, and once all of the dough is rotat-
ing around the edges, count about 10 more revolutions and stop.
Touch the dough. It should be really soft. Let it rest for a full 5 minutes. Put the top back on and process for about 15 more seconds.
Remove the bowl and dump the dough out onto a well-floured surface. Let it rest for about 2 minutes.

Knead the dough with the heels of your hands about 20 times.

Place the dough into a large bowl, cover with plastic wrap, and
allow it to rise in your ideal rising area. If you see butter start to bead
up on the dough, the place you've chosen is too warm. It should take
about an hour for the dough to rise so it is twice as large as it was
when it started.

Deflate the dough by poking your fingers into it. It will return to
a small amount. Turn it out onto your lightly floured surface and pat
it out to a rectangle shape. Fold it in threes back to the original size.
Put the dough back into the bowl, cover, and allow it to rise again so
it is more than double in size.

At this point you can do many different things with the dough:
make loaves, rings, or cinnamon rolls.

To make cinnamon rolls: Make a filling of 1 cup nuts (walnuts,
pecans, etc.), ¾ cup brown sugar, 1 teaspoon cinnamon, ⅛ teaspoon
salt, 1½ cups raisins, and 1 tablespoon corn syrup.

Cut the brioche dough into two parts (you can refrigerate or freeze half for later use). On a floured surface, roll out into a 10 x 14-inch rectangle. Cover this rectangle and chill for about 10 minutes. Remove from refrigerator. Roll the dough out so that it measures about 18 by 12 inches.

Spread the filling over the dough so that it is evenly covered. Starting with one of the long edges, gently roll the dough up to form a long roll. With a very sharp knife slice the log into 10 or 12 portions. Place one roll into each of 12 buttered muffin cups or arrange the slices in a cake pan that has been buttered.

Cover the rolls and allow to rise again for about an hour. They will be very puffy. Bake for about 45 minutes in the middle of a 350° oven. Allow to cool for about 5 minutes and unmold.

$\mathcal{E}$ggs

INCREDIBLY EDIBLE EGGS

*A cook can take a very simple meal, have color in the
menu, a little added flavor in a common dish,
and it looks and tastes gourmet.*
—Paulette Hegg

What is inexpensive, comes neatly sealed in its own unique packaging, contains two distinct and separate components that have vastly different characteristics, and has become a symbol of hope?

An egg is such an ordinary and basic part of life that most of us have never considered its remarkable role in producing a dish extraordinaire. Or a total disaster!

Eggs are more than breakfast food partnered with ham or bacon. When combined with other ingredients, whole eggs, yolks, and whites are critical to a recipe by giving structure, and stability, creating lightness, and blending/binding ingredients that alone are incompatible. They also are responsible for drying or crisping pastries. Never underestimate the importance played by the right amount and condition of eggs in the final outcome of a dish. By getting to know eggs, you'll improve your cooking. Each part of this simple food affects other ingredients in important ways.

The white of an egg is made of protein and water, contains numerous vitamins and minerals, and has only 17 calories. The yolk is made up of fat, cholesterol, and some water; contains more vitamins and minerals, a tiny bit of protein, and about 60 calories. Combined, the yolk and the white form a powerhouse of potent nutrition and contain the highest quality food protein known.

Eggs, both whole and in their separate forms, have many culinary functions. Once you understand what each part of the egg does, you will be able to modify recipes and take better advantage of the particular powers of yolks and whites.

Egg Yolks

Eggs yolks are used to thicken, smooth, and moisten. Because egg yolks contain emulsifiers (the main one being lecithin), they can produce an unbelievably smooth texture. Ingredients that normally would not mix well together blend beautifully and smoothly once an egg yolk has been introduced.

If you have a sauce or caramel that is OK, but not heavenly, consider adding egg yolks.

Egg yolks can thicken and enrich custards, pastry cream, or pie fillings *provided* that once the yolks have been incorporated the mixture is allowed to come to a boil. Here's why: raw egg yolks contain an enzyme called alpha amylase that can destroy a set custard by making it thin and watery. The boiling temperature breaks down the enzyme so that the cooled mixture remains thick and lovely.

Egg Whites

Egg whites dry, repel grease, and give structure. If you need to dry out a dish, add egg whites. If your cream puffs turn out moist and doughy in the center, add an extra egg white for each egg in the recipe and watch them turn out dry and crisp, which is a perfect contrast for the smooth pastry cream made with extra egg yolks.

The uses for whipped egg whites are endless, but there are several things to remember when beating egg whites. First, it is crucial that all of your equipment (beaters, bowl, rubber spatula) be squeaky clean, free of all grease and food particles. Also, the composition of the bowl can make a big difference. Copper bowls react chemically with egg whites to form fluffy, high-rise whites. The same result can be obtained using stainless steel or glass bowls with the addition of cream of tartar. The naturally slick surface of a glass bowl doesn't give as much traction for the egg whites to climb the sides. Never use aluminum (which can cause egg whites to turn slightly gray) or plastic or wooden bowls, which are hard to clean well enough to be fat free.

When deep-frying pieces with batter coating, consider eliminating the yolks from the batter. Yolks absorb grease, while the whites repel it, which will leave your fried batter pieces lighter and not at all greasy.

Buying Eggs

The first rule of eggs: the fresher the better. The very best source of eggs for the gourmet cook is right out of the hen's nest while still warm. The second source for those of us not so fortunate as to have a yard of laying hens is a local egg farm. I live in the middle of a megalopolis yet have fairly convenient access to such a farm where the eggs are always fresh and the prices amazingly low. The source of last resort is the local grocery store and not such a bad one at that, provided you know what to look for and hold out for the best.

If an egg is truly fresh, the white and the yolk cling together tightly when it is cracked open. The older it gets, the flatter the yolk becomes and the more watery the white. Most eggs remain in the fresh state for one week after purchase. Eggs older than this need not be thrown out but are best used in baking and cooking since the fresh flavor has diminished.

The color of an egg's shell has nothing to do with its quality or taste despite common prejudices to the contrary. Buy whichever is cheapest. It's the freshness that is most important. Yolks will vary in color from very pale yellow to golden orange. This color is a result of the chicken's feed and does not make much difference in the taste of the egg.

Storing Eggs

Once an egg is cracked open, its components can be stored for future use. For instance, if you need several egg whites today, the yolks can remain uncooked for two or three days in the refrigerator. Cover them with a film of cold water and plastic wrap to keep a skin from forming. Unbeaten egg whites can be frozen. Egg yolks or whole eggs out of the shell will freeze well provided you add sugar (1 teaspoon per 6 yolks) or salt (½ teaspoon per 6 yolks). Use the sugared eggs in dessert recipes and the salted ones in sauce and egg dishes. Egg whites can be stored in a covered container in the refrigerator for two to three days.

Measuring Eggs

Egg size is standardized by the government. According to those standards a large egg weighs 2 ounces each or 24 ounces for a dozen. A dozen small eggs weigh 18 ounces, and a dozen medium weigh 21 ounces. Extra large eggs are those that weigh 27 ounces to the dozen. One cup of eggs requires 7 small eggs, 6 mediums, 5 large, or 4 extra large. An egg is ⅓ yolk and ⅔ white. A cup of egg whites contains 10 small, 8 medium, 7 large, or 6 extra large egg whites. A cup of egg yolks requires 18 small, 16 medium, 14 large, or 12 extra large egg yolks.

Separating Eggs

Many recipes call for only the white of the egg or just the yolk. It's unfortunate in these cases that whites and yolks come packaged together. However, separating them while leaving both intact is a technique easily mastered by anyone with two clean hands. Plan on spoiling a few eggs before you get the hang of it. Remember that it's easier to separate the white from the yolk when eggs are cold.

Here are the two simplest techniques for separating eggs. Using the first technique, crack the raw egg on the side of a small bowl so that you hold one half of the shell in each hand. While keeping the yolk in one of the shells, allow the white to drip down into the bowl. Now transfer the yolk into the other shell so that more white can drop into the bowl. Keep transferring back and forth until as much white as possible is in the bowl. Transfer the yolk (which by this time should be perfectly whole in one of the shells) into a separate container and discard the shells. If you should break a yolk, start again. A recipe calling for egg whites only may be spoiled by the presence of even the tiniest amount of yolk. The second technique for separating eggs is a little messier but much more reliable. Crack the egg shell and pour its contents into your clean hand that is held over a small bowl. Allow the white to drip between your fingers into the bowl. With a little practice you'll learn to part with all of the white while retaining the intact separated yolk in your hand. Gently deliver it to a second small container.

How to Cook the Perfectly Boiled Egg

A perfectly boiled egg has a yolk that is set all the way to the center and is a clean, beautiful yellow color with no hint of ugly green where the yolk and white meet. A perfectly boiled egg slides smoothly away from the cracked shell.

Prick the shell. Using a push-pin or needle, push it right into the large end of the uncooked egg, in about ¼ inch, and into the egg itself. This will pierce the tiny air bubble (it is present in every egg) that in an unpricked egg expands as the egg is heated and cracks the shell. This tiny hole allows an escape route for the air.

Simmer method. Because this is a tedious process, the maximum number of eggs that should be boiled at one time is twelve. Bring a pot of water to boil. Lower the prepared eggs into the boiling water and bring the water back to a simmer and set the timer: 12 minutes for large chilled eggs and 13 minutes for extra large ones. Keep the water at a low simmer that produces small bubbles and a very slight movement among the eggs.

Coddle method. Some great cooks prefer to coddle eggs rather than simmer because the results are more reliable. Place the chilled eggs in a pot of cold water (6 cups for 1–4 eggs and an additional cup for each additional egg). Bring the water to a full-rolling boil, remove from heat and cover it. Set the timer for exactly 17 minutes (or 18 for jumbo or extra large eggs).

Foolproof peeling of hard-cooked eggs. Tap the egg gently so as to break the shell in many places all around the egg. Start peeling the egg by first placing it under a small stream of cold water and begin removing the shell from the large bottom side. If the shell is resistant and wants to take part of the white with it, simply drop three eggs at a time into boiling water, wait 10 seconds, and immediately transfer them to ice water. This will expand and contract the shell quickly and will release the shell easily.

No more ugly green ring. This change of color occurs when eggs are allowed to remain warm after proper cooking. A chemical reaction between the yolk and the white occurs, causing this discoloration. The way to prevent this is to chill the eggs as quickly as possible. Once the eggs have completed cooking, quickly pour off the hot water and turn a tray of ice into the pan, quickly filling with cold water so they are completely covered.

Store cooked eggs properly. Cooked eggs should be submerged in cold water in an uncovered container and stored in the refrigerator. They will keep for several days this way without loss of flavor, nutrition, or texture.

How to Cook the Perfectly Poached Egg

Reserve poaching for when you have the freshest possible eggs on hand. Fill a sauté, omelet, or frying pan two-thirds of the way with plain water (no vinegar or salt). Bring to a boil. Prick a hole in the large end of each egg as described above. Lower one egg into the water and allow to remain exactly 10 seconds to set the film around the white of the egg. Now carefully break the egg into a flat saucer and carefully slide it into the boiling water. Leave for exactly 4 minutes. With a large slotted spoon, remove the poached egg and transfer it immediately to a bowl of ice water.

Once you have poached the proper number of eggs and are ready to serve them, return them one at a time to the boiling water for exactly 30 seconds. As you remove an egg, set it on a piece of stale bread, which will act as a blotter, then quickly transfer it to your serving plate or pieces of toast.

Poached eggs may be left in the ice water bath and stored in the refrigerator for up to three days. When ready to use, drop them gently into boiling water for exactly 1 minute and proceed as above.

How to Prepare Perfectly Scrambled Eggs

Break 4–6 eggs into a heavy bowl. Add one tablespoon of ice water along with a pinch (or few grinds) of pepper and a pinch of salt. Whip them with a fork just long enough to blend the whites and yolks. (Tip: in scrambled eggs you can get away with using fewer yolks.)

Heat a 10-inch nonstick skillet or sauté pan on a low flame or burner. Melt a tablespoon of butter and pour in all but 2 tablespoons of the whipped egg mixture. After 2 minutes begin scraping the bottom of the pan with a spatula. Slowly the eggs will begin to thicken as you keep scraping more quickly and begin moving the pan back and forth over the burner (this will slow down the cooking). Once the eggs have reached your desired consistency, remove the pan from the heat and stir in the remaining 2 tablespoons of egg. This will help the cooking process to cease and will remoisturize the portions which have become dry. Serve as is, or if you want to dress these eggs up a bit, fold in 2 tablespoons of butter or heavy cream and minced fresh parsley or chives. Serve at once on a warm plate. If you wish to add a sauce, do not stir it in, but instead pour it over the top of the finished eggs.

How to Fry Eggs Perfectly

First preheat your broiler. Next, in a frying pan of a size to accommodate the number of eggs you will be frying, pour in ⅛-inch melted butter, olive oil, or bacon fat. Set the pan over moderately high heat on the stove top and when hot, break in as many as six or eight eggs, being careful not to break the yolks. Cook about one minute (or more) until the white has set nicely on the bottom. Baste the eggs with the fat in the pan, then set the pan closely under the hot broiler. Move the pan back and forth to make sure it is receiving even heat. Baste several times more. Soon the eggs will form a film over the top and will be perfectly cooked both top and bottom with no need to turn.

Tips

♦ Open the carton at the store to check that none of the eggs are cracked. Slightly move each egg with your finger to make sure it isn't stuck to the carton. If after you arrive home you find one or more are stuck, fill the indentations with a little cool water and let stand about 5 minutes. The eggs should loosen easily.

♦ If you're buying eggs to be used in recipes, purchase large eggs. That's what most recipes call for, and the difference between extra-large or medium eggs could significantly alter the outcome.

♦ Always store eggs large end up—it keeps them fresher and helps keep the yolk centered. Also, never store them near pungent foods like onions because they easily absorb odors right through their shells.

♦ When adding eggs to a mixture, break them one at a time into a small bowl. If you break eggs directly into the mixture, you run the risk of spoiling it all with one bad egg.

♦ Dropping an egg on the floor can create a real mess. It'll be easier to clean up if you lightly sprinkle the egg with salt, then let it set for 20 minutes. A damp paper towel will pick the mess right up.

♦ An easy way to freeze extra egg whites is to place one in each section of an ice cube tray. Freeze, then pop the egg white cubes out into a freezer weight plastic bag. Thaw what you need overnight in the refrigerator. They can be stored up to 6 months in the freezer.

♦ When beating egg whites, add a small amount of acid, such as cream of tartar, lemon juice, or vinegar. It stabilizes egg whites and allows them to reach their full volume and stiffness. Use ⅛ teaspoon of the acid ingredient per egg white and add the acid to the whites just as they begin to become frothy during beating.

However, this is not necessary if you are using a copper bowl, as the natural acid on the surface achieves the same result.

♦ When microwaving eggs, yolks cook faster than egg whites because they contain the fat that attracts the microwaves.

♦ Microwave unbeaten eggs at 30 to 40 percent power, beaten egg mixtures at 100 percent power.

How to Test an Egg for Freshness

If an egg floats when submerged in a bowl of water or tips noticeably upward, it means an air sac has expanded and the interior has shrunk away from the shell. The egg is definitely old. It takes at least three weeks for eggs left at room temperature to reach this state, so it is not likely to occur with modern methods of fast distribution and refrigeration. An egg that floats should be discarded.

Some of the Vital Roles Eggs Play in Cooking

Whole Eggs:

Give structure	The proteins in eggs coagulate when heated, forming a resilient but firm web that helps hold together sauces, baked goods, and dishes such as meat loaf.
Leaven	When air is incorporated into eggs by beating (either just a little or a lot, as in eggs beaten to a ribbon stage), the eggs will puff during cooking to leaven or rise whatever they're in.
Glaze and color	Whole eggs, whites, or yolks can be brushed on breads and pastries and baked to give a rich, shiny glaze. Both whites and yolks are high in protein, which encourages browning, so dishes incorporating eggs also take on a deeper golden color.

Egg Yolks:

Bind and thicken   Natural emulsifiers, such as lecithin, hold fat and water together in an emulsion to thicken sauces such as hollandaise and mayonnaise.

Give smoothness   Egg yolks can create a creamy, satiny-smooth texture in everything from chocolate truffles to custards. Their emulsifying power means they bind liquids with fats for sensational smoothness.

Egg Whites:

Dry and crisp   Egg whites contain no fat and can create a dry protein lattice when heated. They help give things like cream puffs a drier, crisper consistency, but too many egg whites in a cake or muffin will make it dry and unpleasant.

Clarify   When mixed with stock and slowly heated, the proteins in egg whites coagulate to trap particles and make the stock crystal clear.

Source: *Fine Cooking Magazine,* April–May 1996, 77.

Broccoli Quiche
Contributed by Deborah Taylor-Hough
6 Servings

Many children do not seem to like quiche, but I have found that what they really are tasting is actually the unusual flavor of the Swiss cheese frequently used in quiche. If you replace Swiss cheese with a combination of Jack and cheddar, kids will eat it up and even ask for seconds!

Crust:
- 2 cups white or brown leftover cooked rice
- 1 egg, beaten
- 1 teaspoon soy sauce

Filling:
- ½ pound broccoli, fresh or frozen, cooked until tender but not soft
- 4 eggs, beaten
- 1½ cups half-and-half (can use milk or cream)
- 1 cup cheese, grated (Swiss, cheddar, Jack, or whatever in any combination)
- salt and pepper to taste
- dash nutmeg or ground mace

Crust: Mix together rice, egg, and soy sauce. Spread evenly to cover well-buttered quiche or pie pan. Bake crust at 350° for 10 minutes. Remove from oven.

Filling: Place broccoli in bottom of crust. Mix together eggs, milk, and spices. Pour over broccoli. Top with cheese. Bake at 350° for 45–50 minutes or until a knife inserted near center of pie comes out clean. Remove from oven and let sit 10 minutes before slicing.

Note: You can use almost any leftover vegetables or meats in this recipe. If you have eggs, milk, and rice, you can practically clean out the refrigerator right into your quiche pan. Just remember to add the cheese last, since it makes a beautiful mellow, brown crust on the top of your pie. (Gourmet has to appeal to the eyes too!)

Nutrient value per serving: 421 calories, 14 g protein, 15 g fat, 57 g carbohydrates, 231 mg sodium, 113 mg cholesterol.

Cheese Strata
8 Servings

5   slices white bread
4   eggs, beaten
2   cups milk
¾   teaspoon brown sugar
¾   teaspoon Worcestershire sauce
¾   teaspoon seasoned salt
¾   teaspoon dry mustard
1   dash white pepper
2½ cups cheddar cheese, shredded

The day before serving, remove crusts and cut bread into cubes. Combine beaten eggs, milk, brown sugar, Worcestershire, seasoned salt, dry mustard, and white pepper in 9 x 13-inch baking dish. Stir in bread and cheese and refrigerate overnight. When ready to cook, bake at 325° for 45 minutes or until knife inserted in center comes out clean.

Nutrient value per serving: 268 calories, 16 g protein, 17 g fat, 13 g carbohydrates, 766 mg sodium, 152 mg cholesterol.

Chili Cheese Strata
6 Servings

5   sourdough bread slices
2   tablespoons butter, softened
8   ounces green chilies, diced or in strips
¾   pound cheddar cheese, shredded
4   eggs
2   tablespoons Dijon mustard
2   cups milk
    salt and pepper to taste

Remove crusts from bread; butter the slices and cut into cubes. Place cubes in an 8 x 8-inch greased baking dish. Cover with cheese and chilies. Whisk together eggs, mustard, milk, salt, and black pepper. Pour over bread cubes. Cover and refrigerate overnight. Bake at 350° for 45 minutes or until nicely brown on top and an inserted knife comes out clean; allow to stand for 10 minutes. Cut into 4-inch squares and serve with salsa and sour cream.

Nutrient value per serving: 443 calories, 25 g protein, 30 g fat, 19 g carbohydrates, 719 mg sodium, 223 mg cholesterol.

Elegant Quiche
6 Servings

Pastry crust:

2	cups flour
1	dash salt
1	cup butter
1	tablespoon oil
2 to 4	tablespoons cold water

1	onion, chopped
1	tablespoon butter
1	dash thyme
1	bay leaf
5	ounces bacon, chopped
5	eggs
2	egg yolks
1	cup half-and-half
1	dash nutmeg
⅓	pound Swiss cheese, shredded

Pastry shell: Mix flour and salt together in bowl. Cut in butter and oil until mixture resembles coarse meal. Sprinkle with water, tossing with fork until dough holds together. Gather into a ball and chill a few minutes if dough is too soft to handle. Roll out pastry on floured board and fit into 10-inch quiche pan or pie plate.

Sauté onion in butter. Add thyme and bay leaf. Remove bay leaf. Cook bacon until crisp, then drain. Blend together eggs, yolks, half-and-half, and nutmeg. Place bacon, onion, and cheese in pastry shell. Cover with egg mixture. Bake at 350° for 35 to 40 minutes or until knife inserted near center comes out clean.

Nutrient value per serving: 493 calories, 22 g protein, 28 g fat, 38 g carbohydrates, 359 mg sodium, 301 mg cholesterol.

Frittata
8 Servings

  2 small eggplants, thinly sliced
  ½ teaspoon salt
  ½ cup olive oil
  2 baking potatoes, peeled and thinly sliced
  1 large onion, peeled and thinly sliced
  2 small zucchinis, thinly sliced
  1 red pepper, minced
 12 eggs
     salt, to taste
     pepper, to taste
     fresh thyme, sprigs to taste

Preheat oven to 450°. Sprinkle ½ teaspoon salt over the eggplant slices. Place slices into a colander or strainer and allow to sit for about 10 minutes. Rinse with cold water, spread on a clean towel, and pat them dry. Pour olive oil into a 9 x 18 inch baking dish. Place in oven and heat for about 5 minutes and remove. Arrange potato and onion slices in baking dish and bake for 20 minutes or until potatoes are slightly tender. Arrange the zucchini and eggplant slices on top of the potatoes and onions. Bake for another 5 minutes. Sprinkle the red pepper (make sure it's a sweet red bell pepper and not a chili pepper) over the other vegetables. Beat the eggs and season with salt and pepper. Pour the eggs over the vegetables and arrange the thyme on top. Bake until the eggs are set and the sides have puffed, about 20 minutes. Reduce oven temperature if eggs appear to be cooking too fast. The top will become golden brown, and a knife inserted in the middle should come out clean. Do not overcook. The frittata should be firm but not dry. Cut into squares and serve hot or at room temperature.

Nutrient value per serving: 333 calories, 12 g protein, 23 g fat, 19 g carbohydrates, 392 mg sodium, 319 mg cholesterol.

Italian Eggs
8 Servings

This is an excellent choice for brunch or Christmas morning.

8 slices white bread, cubed
1½ pounds sweet Italian sausage, broken up
¾ pounds cheddar cheese, grated
4 eggs
2 cups milk
¾ teaspoon dry mustard
1 6½ ounce can cream of mushroom soup
1 4 ounce can sliced, drained mushrooms

Butter a 9 x 13-inch dish. Line dish with bread cubes like a shell. Brown the sausage; discard grease. Put sausage and cheese in shell. In a small bowl, beat the eggs with milk and mustard. Pour over all. Refrigerate, covered overnight. Just before baking combine soup and mushrooms and pour over dish. Bake at 325° for 1½ hours.

Nutrient value per serving: 511 calories, 30 g protein, 34 g fat, 20 g carbohydrates, 981 mg sodium, 203 mg cholesterol.

Chapter 10

Meats, Fish, and Seafood

LUXURIES FROM THE TURF TO THE SURF

You may be extraordinarily creative and imaginative in the kitchen, but you cannot take advantage of these qualities if you do not know the basics.
—Jacques Pépin

Americans have long been, and undoubtedly will continue to be, big meat-eaters. While some nutritional schools of thought have suggested that the total elimination of meat from one's diet would be a wise move, others disagree vehemently, encouraging a diet high in animal protein. With the results of nutritional education so readily available, many of us in the last decade are eating less meat. However, Americans still manage to consume more meat per capita than any other country in the world. Our meals are typically planned around meat, and meat consumes more of the average family's food dollar than anything else we eat.

In that it would be impossible to go into a meaningful discussion on the grades and specific cuts of all meats, there is a booklet you should have in your kitchen library on this subject, and I highly recommend you order a copy of it immediately. *Confessions of a Butcher: Eat Steak on a Hamburger Budget and Save* by John Smith is designed specifically for us, the home cooks. It contains photographs, names, and pictures of all standard cuts of meat along with descriptions and basic cooking methods. At this writing the cost is $5.95 plus $2.00 shipping/handling and can be obtained by writing: Ark Essentials, P.O. Box 12062, Salem, OR 07309. Not only will this equip you with valuable information, it will also give you confidence in venturing out into preparing and serving different cuts of meat.

Buying Ground Meat

Whether it is ground beef, veal, lamb, or pork, ground meat is one of the most economical food buys in the meat market. When buying ground beef (or any cut of beef), look for brightly colored, red to deep red cuts. You will be confronted with a wide range of choices from which to select. Labels such as hamburger, ground beef, ground chuck, ground round, and ground sirloin do little more than confuse the shopper.

When it comes to ground meat, the price generally reflects the quality and the market where the meat is purchased, whether supermarket or specialty butcher. The higher the fat content, the lower the price. However, remember that fat greatly contributes to flavor, and the lower the fat content, the drier the cooked meat will be. Even if fat content is an important consideration for you, high-fat meat might still be an option when making dishes that require the meat to be browned, such as meatballs. That way, much of the fat will cook out of the meat and can be drained off.

Ground meat is generally ground from less tender cuts of meat. However, this doesn't affect its nutritional value since tender and less tender cuts of meat contain about the same amount of protein, vitamins, and minerals. For this reason ground meat is one of the most economical as well as nutritional buys.

Herbs to Use with Meat

Heighten the flavor of ground meat with the addition of herbs and spices. By using just the right seasoning, you can transform an acceptable food into a mouthwatering dish. Some familiar seasonings often added to beef include chili powder, garlic, mustard, and oregano. For a change of pace, add basil, cumin, curry, dill, marjoram, savory, or thyme to beef. Accent veal with basil, curry, ginger, mace, marjoram, mustard, sage, or savory. Lamb is a natural with mint, oregano, rosemary, savory, or thyme. Try blending the subtle flavor of pork with clove, ginger, garlic, mustard, oregano, sage, or thyme. Pair ham with allspice, cinnamon, clove, ginger, or mustard. Sausage may not need additional seasoning, but if mildly seasoned, flavor with garlic, oregano, sage, or thyme.

Cooking Ground Meat

Recent discovery of deadly bacteria have changed the way we think of and prepare ground meats. Gone are the days when one could confidently serve raw ground meat dishes (such as steak tartar) or offer rare hamburgers. *Without exception* all ground meat must be cooked to an interior temperature of not less than 155°. This means hamburgers should be ordered and prepared well done. Period. No exceptions.

However, before your mouth dries up thinking about shoe leather on a bun, there are ways to rescue, resuscitate, and make mouthwatering, well-cooked hamburgers. It's all in the preparation. Try adding a half cup of barbecue sauce, ketchup, tomato or vegetable juice, beef broth, or other liquid to a pound of ground beef, along with seasonings and chopped onions. Or stuff your ground meat with cheese and minced leftover veggies. You will not only have moist mouthwatering burgers, but they are very gourmet and perfect for that special outdoor dinner party. Let's face it; it doesn't matter how old we are, or how sophisticated the palate, everyone loves a great burger every once in a while.

Freezing and Storing Ground Meat

The versatility of ground meat makes it an excellent food to have on hand for quick meals or unexpected dinner guests. Its shelf life in comparison to other foods, however, is quite short unless it is properly wrapped and refrigerated. Ground meat is more perishable than steaks, roasts, or chops since it has been ground, thus exposing more of the surface area of the meat to the air. Consequently, unless a freezer is available, only the amount of ground meat that can be used within two days should be purchased at one time.

To ensure maximum freshness and quality of ground meat as it is purchased, remove store wrappings and rewrap loosely in plastic wrap or a plastic bag immediately after purchasing. Store in the coldest part of the refrigerator to use within two days. In the freezer, storage time for ground meat may be lengthened up to two or three months. Wrap tightly in moisture vapor-proof material such as freezer paper or plastic bags. Seal; label with the name of contents, date, and the amount. Freeze at zero degrees or below. Ground meat works well when prepared before freezing. If you should see a great bargain on meat that is nearing its expiration date, purchase only if you will be able to brown all of it, divide in usable portions, and freeze for future use.

Shaping Ground Meat

For ground meat products that are juicy and light, the trick is to handle the meat as little as possible. Too much handling gives ground meat a compact texture. This is the last thing you want in meat loaves, patties, or meatballs.

Meats for Sautés

Sautéing is the quickest and easiest way to cook a steak or chop, and it has the happy advantage of practically making its own simple and delicious sauce from the juices left in the pan (deglaze with chicken, beef, or vegetable stock). Cuts that lend themselves to sauté preparation are steaks, pork and veal chops, veal scallops, ham steaks, calves' liver, and hamburgers.

Meats for Roasting

Roast beef usually means roast ribs of beef and, like the traditional turkey, is one of the easiest pieces to prepare. Set it in the oven on a rack over a roasting pan, baste it occasionally, and watch the meat thermometer, which should be placed so the strip is embedded in the center or thickest part of the cut. A roast can be held perfectly for up to an hour. While many cuts of meat can be roasted acceptably, the traditional roasting choices are ribs, top loin, tenderloin, and roast leg of lamb, roast pork, and ham shoulder.

Every well-rounded cook should have in his or her repertoire the recipes and experience in preparing the basic four impressive meat dinners. You know, the meals that everyone oohs and ahhs over. They are the roast prime rib of beef, roast leg of lamb or rack of lamb, roast leg of fresh pork, and a braised whole ham. If you master these, your reputation as a fabulous cook will quickly spread far and wide. The key is not to be intimidated by the elegant nature of these dishes, realizing that most of the work is done by your oven. I recommend you do as I have done and once again let Julia be your personal coach. In *The Way to Cook* (Alfred A. Knopf, 1989) she has what she calls "master recipes" wherein she takes great care to explain how to prepare, in this case, roasted meats.

Pot Roasts, Braised Meats, Stews, and Ragouts

These are the tougher (and therefore cheaper) cuts of meat that do best when simmered in quality tasting liquids with onions, herbs, and other good things. A beef pot roast is half the price of the top loin roast, for instance. These tougher cuts are generally more flavorful than their expensive roasting cousins and require long, slow, moist cooking. Whether it's going to be called a pot roast, stew, ragout, or braised beef, the process is the same: first the meat is browned, then it is simmered in a fragrant liquid.

Seafood

While quality species of fish are becoming more and more expensive, if you are fortunate to catch your own or live in an area where supply and demand reward you with bargains, you are indeed fortunate and should take every advantage of knowing how to prepare them perfectly.

Freshness is the cardinal rule when it comes to the enjoyment of fresh fish. Your nose will always be the best judge. If it smells "fishy," has a chemical quality, or is not just right, it's not fresh, and the best advice is to pass. Fresh fish can be held for a few days in the refrigerator provided you immediately place the chilled fish in a plastic bag, enclose that in another plastic bag, set them in a bowl with ice cubes, and place in the refrigerator. Be certain to renew the ice often. Even frozen fish should have a pleasant smell when it thaws. Frozen fish must be handled well. Never thaw on a countertop or in the sink but in the refrigerator.

Fish Can Be Broiled, Braised, or Roasted

The method of cooking depends not only on its size and thickness but the effect you're after. Thin fillets are best broiled two to three minutes under the broiler. Thick fillets and steaks need different treatment and are excellent for other cooking possibilities.

Timing the Cooking of Fish

The rule of timing fish is ten minutes per inch at the thickest portion. However, keep in mind that every rule has its exception, so start checking for doneness after seven minutes. Always cut into the fish to check its doneness. The flesh should be firm and not opaque, but solid salmon-colored or white.

Cooking Methods

For moist-heat cooking methods like poaching, steaming, or stewing, choose lean fish fillets ¼- to ⅜-inch thick such as cod, flounder, perch, red snapper, or sole. For dry-heat cooking methods like baking, broiling, and grilling, choose moderate- to high-fat fish such as bluefish, butterfish, catfish, salmon, striped bass, swordfish, or trout.

For fat-based cooking methods like sautéing, pan-frying, or deep-frying, lean to moderate-fat fish are the best choice; lean fish can also be used. High-fat fish are too rich to fry. When pan frying, don't bread fish too far in advance, or it will become soggy. Pan searing in a hot skillet seals in the rich juices, and it is one of the easiest ways to prepare salmon, for example. Warm the pan before you add the oil, which allows the pan to get really hot without burning the oil. A preheated pan also requires less oil. Simply cook the salmon until golden brown on the bottom (about 4 minutes), turn the salmon and lower the heat to moderate and sear until just cooked (3–4 minutes longer). This method also works well for other meaty fish or even sea scallops.

If you cook a lot of fish, invest in a wide (5–6 inches) slotted spatula for transferring fish from pan to plate.

Fish needs insulation in order to stay moist while baking. The baking dish can be covered, or the fish itself coated with butter and crumbs or topped with a sauce before being baked. Lean fish such as flounder or halibut can be covered with a layer of finely chopped vegetables, herbs, etc. Baking fish at 450° will quickly seal in the fish's natural juices, making it deliciously moist and tender.

To cook a whole fish, size determines the preparation and cooking time. When roasting a whole fish of about one pound, remember to dredge in flour so as to crisp the skin during cooking and discourage it from sticking to the roasting pan. Larger fish like bass or salmon don't need dredging but do take about double the time in the oven.

The French technique of wrapping fish in parchment paper or foil (en papillote) is the perfect way to keep baked fish moist. Cut a piece of parchment paper or foil large enough to enclose the fish, butter the paper or foil, and lay the seasoned fish on top. Bring paper or foil over the top of the fish; roll or fold the edges to seal the package tightly. Bake 7 to 10 minutes per inch of thickness. To serve, place the package directly on a plate, slash an X in the top and peel back the paper or foil.

Barbecuing

Building a Fire for Barbecue:

◆ Start fire 45 minutes to 1 hour before actual cooking is to begin.

◆ Use charcoal briquettes for an even, intense fire.

◆ To kindle, start with a few rolls of newspaper or kindling wood. Fan flames to keep fire burning. Burn coals until they are glowing and coated with white ashes. Don't cook over flames, or food will burn.

◆ Use the heat remaining in the coals after the main meal is cooked to toast marshmallows, grill banana chunks, pop popcorn, etc.

◆ Cleanup will be easier if you coat the grill with nonstick vegetable spray before beginning to cook. Don't spray the grill over the fire or you could have a flare-up.

◆ Wood chips add a wonderful smokiness to grilled foods. Mesquite lends a delicate, sweeter nuance than the more intense (but still sweet) hickory. Try other woods such as apple, cherry, maple, peach, pecan, and walnut. Always soak wood chips in water for an hour before using, wood chunks for 2 hours. Drain thoroughly before sprinkling over hot coals.

◆ Dried herbs such as oregano, tarragon, or rosemary sprinkled over hot coals just before grilling add fragrance and flavor to food.

◆ Remove food from the grill a minute or two before it's done—the residual heat will continue to cook the food.

Preparing Meats and Seafood for Barbecuing:

◆ Thaw meat in refrigerator or in microwave—never on the countertop.

◆ Thoroughly wash hands before handling food and again after handling meat.

◆ Turn your steaks with tongs or a spatula—a fork pierces the meat and causes juices to escape.

◆ For an uncomplicated, great-tasting barbecued entrée, soak flank steak in soy sauce for 3–4 hours. Cook on very hot grill for 7–8 minutes on the first side and 6–7 minutes on the other. Slice thinly on the bias.

- Salt your steaks after cooking—salt draws the juices out.
- Cook hamburger until no pink juices are visible. Use a clean and sanitized temperature probe to make sure burgers are cooked to an internal temperature of 155°.
- Turn patties over at least once.
- To keep in juices, do not press patties with spatula.
- Leave the skin on fish fillets to be grilled, and they'll retain their shape better. If desired, remove the skin after cooking.
- Marinate meat in plastic food-storage bags or glass, ceramic, or stainless steel containers. Most marinades contain acids, which can react with metal and affect the flavor.
- Don't place grilled food back on the same platter it was on when it was raw. Wash the platter after it has held raw meat, or use a separate plate for serving grilled food.
- Boil marinade or basting sauce used with raw meat at least three minutes before serving it alongside the cooked food. Otherwise dispose of marinade.
- Eat burgers immediately or refrigerate them. Do not let patties stand at room temperature.
- Prepared mayonnaise generously smeared on fish fillets and fish steaks will prevent them from sticking when they are barbecued. Most of the mayonnaise will cook off, leaving the fish moist and tasty.
- Grill twice as much fish as you need for dinner, cover, and refrigerate the leftovers to be used the next day in a cold fish salad.

Turning Boring Burgers into Gourmet Delights:

- Before forming into patties, add different spices to the meat: garlic powder, dry soup mix, chili powder, oregano.
- Try a different type of bread for the bun: French roll, pumpernickel, Hawaiian sweet bread, cinnamon bread, garlic or basil rolls.
- Toppings individualize a burger: avocado, pineapple, green chili slices, fried or scrambled egg, peanut butter, wine cheese, sliced cucumbers, spinach.

◆ Sauces add variety too—hot mustard, ranch salad dressing, Italian dressing, garlic paste, barbecue sauce.
◆ Add a stiffly beaten egg to the mixture after you've seasoned it. The cooked burgers will be light and juicy.

Broiling

Broiling is a very controlled method of cooking meat and seafood, as it is so fast. The key to broiling either meat or seafood is to choose fish fillets or steaks that are about 1 inch thick. Thicker than that and the exterior can char before the inside is done. Thinner will too quickly produce well-done disks.

Broiled meat, fish, or poultry will brown more evenly if brought to room temperature before cooking. Position steak or fillet so that the top surface is 3 to 6 inches from the heat source. The thicker the cut, the greater the distance. If broiling fish, there's usually no need to turn it. The radiant heat will cook it through. The general rule, however, is that the longer the fish or meat cooks, the tougher it gets.

When fish steaks are more than ¾ inch thick, use the broil roast method so that the fish will cook evenly. Brown the top nicely under the broiler and finish by baking at 375° in the upper third of the oven, basting occasionally with the juices in the dish.

Tips

◆ Make cleanup easy by spraying the broiler pan with nonstick vegetable spray before beginning to cook.
◆ Broiled meat, fish, or poultry will brown more evenly if brought to room temperature before cooking.
◆ Think of expensive meats and fish as flavorings rather than the star attraction. Build dinners around less costly pastas or grains.
◆ Use intense tastes like flavored canned tomatoes as penny-wise oomph for meat.
◆ Double the vegetables and halve the meat when making kabobs.
◆ Tea can be used as a meat tenderizer, particularly for stew meat. In a Dutch oven, sear chunks of stew meat in fat or oil until very

well browned. Add 2 cups strong black tea, bring to a boil, then cover and simmer for 30 minutes. Add stock and continue to cook stew with additional ingredients as usual.

♦ It's easier to slice meat thinly for quick-cooking dishes like stir fry if you first freeze the meat for 30–60 minutes.

♦ When buying fresh, whole fish, look for bright, clear, full eyes; shiny, brightly colored skin; firm flesh that springs back when pressed with your finger; a fresh mild odor; and red to bright pink gills that are free of slime or residue. Fish fillets and steaks should have a fresh odor, firm texture, and moist appearance.

♦ Before handling fish, rinse your hands in cold water, and they won't smell as fishy.

♦ Tweezers are perfect for removing fine bones from cooked fish.

Blue Bayou Monte Cristo Sandwich
1 Serving

A tasty Southern specialty, this makes an everyday sandwich into an occasion. The light egg batter appeals to just about everyone and gives the dish a delightfully different twist.

Batter:
1½ cups all-purpose flour, sifted
¼ teaspoon salt
1 tablespoon baking powder
1⅓ cups water
1 egg

Sandwich:
¾ ounce turkey, sliced
¾ ounce Swiss cheese, sliced
¾ ounce ham, sliced
2 slices egg bread
canola oil for deep-frying

Batter directions: Sift flour, salt, and baking powder together. Add water to beaten egg, then add to flour mixture and mix well. Set aside.

Make a sandwich using turkey first, then swiss cheese, then ham. Cut sandwich into quarters diagonally using toothpicks to hold sandwich together. Dip sandwich sections in egg batter and fry in 360° canola oil until golden brown. Remove toothpicks and sprinkle with powdered sugar. Arrange four quarters on each serving plate. Serve with raspberry or strawberry jam. Yum.

Nutrient value per serving: 1,061 calories, 45 g protein, 18 g fat, 1,180 g carbohydrates, 2,310 mg sodium, 259 mg cholesterol.

Broiled Steak and Béarnaise Sauce
2 Servings

- 2 12-ounce sirloin tip steaks
- 1 tablespoon unsalted butter
- ¼ cup red wine vinegar
- ¼ cup chicken stock
- 1½ tablespoons shallots, minced
- ½ tablespoon dried tarragon
-     salt and pepper, to taste
- 3 egg yolks
- 1 tablespoon lemon juice
- 1 stick unsalted butter, melted
- 2 tablespoons fresh tarragon, minced (or parsley)

Preheat broiler. To make the sauce, boil vinegar, stock, shallots, dried tarragon, and salt and pepper in a small saucepan until reduced to about 2 tablespoons. Strain in a sieve, reserving the liquid, and cool. Whisk together egg yolks, lemon juice, and reserved liquid in a small bowl, or place these ingredients in a blender and mix at high speed. Slowly pour a steady stream of melted butter as you continue whisking, or if using a blender, as it runs. When all is well blended, pour sauce into a bowl. Stir in minced herbs and correct seasonings by tasting the finished sauce. Set aside. Put steaks on a broiler rack and broil on each side for exactly 5 minutes. The steaks will be rare. Dot the steaks with butter, season to taste, and serve immediately with béarnaise sauce.

Nutrient value per serving: 753 calories, 78 g protein, 43 g fat, 4 g carbohydrates, 772 mg sodium, 533 mg cholesterol.

Ginger-Mustard Salmon with Lemon Sauce
4 Servings

Marinade:
1   piece fresh ginger, about a 1-inch cube, peeled
1   teaspoon lemon zest
3   tablespoons lemon juice
3   tablespoons vegetable oil
2   tablespoons honey
2   teaspoons Dijon mustard
2   teaspoons soy sauce
½   teaspoon salt
4   salmon fillets, about 6 to 7 ounces each

Sauce:
1   tablespoon seasoned rice vinegar
½   cup chicken stock
1   shallot, minced
1   teaspoon dried rosemary
3   tablespoons whipping cream
2   tablespoons unsalted butter, cold
    salt, and freshly ground white pepper to taste
    fresh chives, optional

For the marinade, mince ginger with lemon zest in a food processor or blender. Add lemon juice, 2 tablespoons of the oil, honey, mustard, soy sauce, and salt; mix well. Reserve half of the marinade to use for the sauce. Transfer the rest to a large plastic food bag and add salmon. Refrigerate at least 30 minutes or as long as 8 hours.

Heat oven to 450°. Heat remaining oil in a heavy, ovenproof skillet, preferably cast-iron, over high heat. Add salmon, skin side down, and cook 3 minutes. Transfer to the oven, cook just until cooked through, about 5 to 6 minutes.

Begin the sauce while the salmon is cooking. Combine chicken stock, vinegar, shallot, and rosemary in a small nonaluminum pan. Boil over high heat until it is reduced to 3 tablespoons, 6 to 8 minutes. Add reserved marinade and cream. Turn heat to low. Cut the butter into 2 pieces. Whisk them in one at a time, waiting until the first piece is incorporated before adding the other. Add salt and pepper to taste. Sauce can be made a day ahead and gently reheated on the stove top or using medium (50 percent) power in the microwave oven.

Strain sauce over fish. Garnish with chives, if desired.

Nutrient value per serving: 606 calories, 47 g protein, 9 g fat, 12 g carbohydrates, 682 mg sodium, 179 mg cholesterol.

Imperial Flank Steak
8 Servings

2   pounds flank steak, tenderized once by butcher
½   cup brown sugar, packed
½   cup soy sauce
1   teaspoon garlic powder
1   teaspoon ground ginger
5   eggs, beaten
1   bunch green onion tops, chopped
    cornstarch
    oil

Cut steak into bite-size pieces. In large bowl stir together brown sugar, soy sauce, garlic powder, and ginger. Add flank steak and marinate 15 minutes. Combine eggs and green onions in medium bowl. Place cornstarch in separate bowl. Dip each piece of meat lightly into cornstarch. Dip into beaten egg mixture.

Heat ½-inch oil in medium-sized skillet. Fry meat in hot oil until golden brown, turning once. Drain on paper towels and serve with steamed white rice.

Nutrient value per serving: 275 calories, 28 g protein, 13 g fat, 10 g carbohydrates, 1,142 mg sodium, 190 mg cholesterol.

Mexicali Fish
4 Servings

¼ cup cornmeal
¼ cup flour
1 pinch salt and pepper
4 5 ounce fish fillets, ¾ inch thick
2 tablespoons oil
⅓ cup sour cream
2 tablespoons green chilies, chopped
⅓ cup Monterey Jack cheese, shredded
     fresh parsley, chopped
     paprika

Combine cornmeal, flour, salt, and black pepper. Dredge fish in cornmeal mixture. Place fish in an oiled skillet and fry over medium high until golden brown on each side, about 5 minutes per side or until fish begins to flake easily. Combine sour cream, chilies, and cheese. Pour over fish and place 6 inches below a preheated broiler. Broil 3 minutes or until lightly browned. Sprinkle with parsley and paprika for color.

Nutrient value per serving: 266 calories, 34 g protein, 8 g fat, 14 g carbohydrates, 740 mg sodium, 86 mg cholesterol.

Sea Scallops with Garlic and Herbs
6 Servings

1½ pounds scallops, cleaned and cut into thirds
      salt and freshly ground pepper
½   cup flour, for dredging
¼   cup clarified butter
1   clove garlic, minced
1½ tablespoons scallions, minced
      minced fresh parsley for garnish

Dry the scallops and spread them out on a sheet of waxed paper. Toss them with a little salt and pepper. Heat clarified butter in a large sauté pan. Right before scallops go into the pan, dredge them in the flour, place them in a sieve, and shake off the excess flour. Pop into hot butter over high heat. Let them sit for just a few seconds and then begin tossing and swirling until scallops brown slightly. Toss in the garlic and scallions. Add the parsley and toss a bit longer. The whole operation should last about 3 to 4 minutes. Serve at once.

Nutrient value per serving: 259 calories, 34 g protein, 9 g fat, 11 g carbohydrates, 391 mg sodium, 89 mg cholesterol.

Swiss and "Crab" Quiche
Contributed by Deborah Taylor-Hough
6 Servings

Crust:
2 cups cooked rice, white or brown (use leftovers!)
1 egg, beaten
1 teaspoon soy sauce

Filling:
2 green onions, sliced with tops
4 ounces Swiss cheese, shredded
8 ounces imitation crab, OR one 7½ ounce can crab meat, drained and flaked
4 eggs, beaten
1½ cups light cream or milk
½ teaspoon salt
½ teaspoon lemon peel, grated
¼ teaspoon dry mustard
1 dash nutmeg or ground mace
⅛ cup sliced almonds

Crust: Mix together rice, egg, and soy sauce. Spread evenly to cover well-buttered quiche or pie pan. Bake crust at 350° for 10 minutes. Remove from oven.

Filling: Arrange cheese on bottom of rice pie shell. Top with crab meat. Sprinkle with green onions. Mix together eggs, milk, salt, lemon peel, mustard, and nutmeg. Pour evenly over top of quiche. Sprinkle almonds over top. Bake at 325° for 45 minutes or until set. Remove from oven and let sit for 10 minutes before slicing.

Note to cheapskates: I have received just as many compliments on this dish when I use the imitation crabmeat as when I use the real thing. It just plain tastes good, either way, and it looks really pretty with the almonds and green onions on top. If you are a purist and cannot fathom the idea of using "fake fish," I often find canned crab on sale for less than $2 a can. That's a great price considering I've seen it as high as $6 a can at my local grocery store. Watch the ads and stock up. I try to keep the ingredients for this quiche on hand at all times. This meal is very light, simple, and goes together quickly, so it's great for spur-of-the-moment luncheons or unexpected guests.

Nutrient value per serving: 418 calories, 16 g protein, 28 g fat, 27 g carbohydrates, 660 mg sodium, 162 mg cholesterol.

Chapter 11

$\mathcal{P}$oultry and Wild Game

WILD THING, YOU MAKE MY HEART SING!

A gourmet meal is in some way unique.
—Bob Kingsbury

Poultry is a generic term for any domesticated bird used for food, the most common being chicken, rock Cornish game hen, and turkey. When purchasing poultry, look for the meaty, full-breasted specimen. A scrawny bird means you're paying for a lot of bone and little meat. The skin should be smooth and soft, not bruised or torn. The younger the bird, the more tender the meat and the milder the flavor. The pinker the bone ends, the fresher the bird. Avoid poultry with an off odor. If buying prepackaged poultry, make sure the cellophane isn't torn and that the package isn't leaking. Check the expiration date on the label to be sure the bird isn't past its prime.

Poultry should be stored in the coldest spot in the refrigerator at 40° or below. Raw poultry can be refrigerated for up to two days; cooked poultry up to three days.

Freezing poultry causes it to lose a lot of the natural juices and can create toughness of the flesh. If you have to freeze poultry, seal it airtight in a freezer-proof plastic bag or foil. When thawing poultry, do so in the refrigerator, not on the countertop.

Commercial salad dressing makes an easy, instant marinade for all kinds of poultry. My favorite is a balsamic vinegar Italian dressing.

162

CAUTION: Bacteria on raw poultry can contaminate other food it comes in contact with, so it's vital you always use hot, soapy water to thoroughly wash your hands, cutting board, and any utensils used in the preparation of poultry. Never let any raw juices come in contact with cooked poultry.

Despite the precautions cooks need to take, poultry, most commonly chicken and turkey, continues to be popular with both the home and professional cook. Entire cooking sections in bookstores are filled with cookbooks for poultry. It is one of those wonderful foods that transcends all meals, from a chicken omelet for breakfast, turkey fajitas for lunch, and blackened chicken for dinner. Poultry can be prepared in any form using any heating method and can be served warm or cold. Not many foods can lay claim to that. Couple that with the dire warnings by nutrition experts about the dangers of eating red meat, and chicken and turkey have been placed atop the food pedestal.

The most wonderful part is that poultry is so economical both in terms of cost and methods of use. A whole chicken is always cheaper than a cut-up one, and a whole chicken can be cooked and used for soups, salads, cassoulets, pastas, and most ethnic dishes.

Learn how to cut a chicken yourself, and you'll be able to spend less in the poultry section. A good pair of poultry shears will help immensely in breaking through joints, cutting through skin, and making the task as neat and quick as possible. After a while you'll get so good at this you can start buying several chickens at a time and cutting them up and freezing similar parts for various recipes. Pretty soon you'll have quite a supply of every cook's favorite: the skinless, boneless chicken breast—you know, the one that costs an arm and a leg in the grocery store.

For the cook who wants to prepare something that everyone likes, is easy to fix, and lets your imagination run wild, chicken breasts are for you. You can bake, broil, grill, poach, and fry them, and the only thing to remember is that they don't take very long to cook. What could be simpler! But regardless of whether you take a fancy to preparing chicken breasts, cooking poultry will result in satisfied dinner guests as long as you pay close attention to how long it's supposed to cook.

When poultry is properly cooked to doneness, the juices run clear, and the meat near the bone at the thickest part is no longer pink. Drumsticks should twist easily in their sockets. Always allow poultry to rest for a few minutes after it's finished cooking to allow the juices to redistribute throughout the flesh, and the meat will be more moist than if carved immediately after cooking.

For those of you who feel accomplished, and perhaps a bit bored with chicken and turkey, don't forget about those wonderful little "mini" turkeys, the Cornish game hen. With more attention paid to them during the holiday season, game hens are often the forgotten member of the poultry family. However, because they are normally sold frozen, they are a good item to stock up on during sales, as they are more expensive than chicken. If you've ever served game hens at any kind of family gathering or dinner party, the feedback is always the same, the presentation on the plate is impressive, and the taste is out of this world. And because everyone gets his own hen, serving is a snap because you, the cook, don't have to deal with any of the carving or serving. And you don't have to guess how many pounds will feed a particular number of people. Recipes abound for stuffings and sauces for game hens, and most of your favorites for turkey or chicken can be adapted to accompany hens, as well.

Wild Game

Other members of the poultry family, not as common as the previously mentioned three, are duck and goose. That's right, they're birds and definitely related to the others. Chicken, turkey, and game hens share similar flavors and textures, but prepared goose has crisp brown skin and all dark meat. It's not a tender bird like chicken and has a certain texture, chewiness, and special flavor all its own. However, the problem with goose is fat. Duck shares this problem (although unlike goose, duck does have perfect breast meat), and as such, both require a bit more attention while cooking.

First the duck or goose should be steamed for about an hour on top of the stove. This takes out a great deal of the fat. Then it should be braised in a covered roaster with aromatic flavorings for another hour or so at 325°. This renders out even more fat. Finally it is left uncovered to brown for about half an hour to let the skin brown and crisp. In Julia Child's *The Way to Cook*, she takes us step-by-step through the process of cooking goose and duck.

For those cooks who have an ongoing supply of wild fowl such as pheasant, we are happy to oblige you with several recipes at the end of this chapter, supplied by our panelists. Though city folks may not have pheasant readily available, these young birds can be used in any recipe for chicken, and vice versa. I will not go into detail here about what one does after acquiring a pheasant from nature, other than to say it's a lot more work than picking up a chicken from the grocery store—but well worth the effort.

Tips

♦ Dry spots on frozen fowl can and usually do mean freezer burn. Smell carefully, and if you have any doubts, return it or toss it. If it smells all right, rub the skin with oil just before roasting.

♦ It is easier to cut cooked or raw birds with scissors, as with cooked chicken or turkey; it doesn't shred the meat as much as a knife.

♦ Meat tenderizers work well with fowl. For poultry cooked in liquid, add a pinch of baking soda to the liquid. For broiling or roasting, rub throughout with lemon juice before cooking.

♦ Cooked poultry can get so dry, especially turkey. To save your guests the ordeal of a dry meal, slice the turkey and arrange on a heat-proof platter. Prepare a sauce of half butter and half chicken broth. Pour it on the sliced bird, and let it stand in a 250° oven for 10 minutes to soak up the juices.

♦ Out of string to truss the bird? Try using unflavored dental floss.

♦ White meat cooks more quickly than dark meat, so if you're cooking pieces, add the white meat portions about five minutes after the rest.

♦ When grilling or broiling, leave the skin on during cooking. It keeps the juices in and creates a more tender result. Remove the skin after the dish is cooked.

- Put all bones in a large pot, cover with water, and bring to a boil. Reduce heat, cover, and simmer for one hour. Cool to room temperature, strain, then refrigerate or freeze for use in soups, stews, sauces, and the like.
- You can use two small birds if four people insist on drumsticks. This will also provide more of the other pieces and a shorter cooking time.
- Plastic cooking bags can reduce a bird's cooking time and produce a beautifully browned bird.
- Birds will almost baste themselves if you cover them with a double layer of cheesecloth that's been soaked with butter or canola or olive oil. When the cheesecloth is removed at the end of the roasting time, the bird will be moist and golden brown. For a crisp, brown skin, take off the cheesecloth 30 minutes before the bird is done.
- Since many recipes call for cooked chicken, here are the equivalents: a 3 to 4 pound broiler-fryer will yield about 3 to 4 cups of cooked chicken, after deboning. A ¾-pound skinned, deboned chicken breast will yield about 2 cups of cooked chicken.
- Rubbing mayonnaise all over the skin produces a crisp, deep golden brown roasted chicken or turkey. However, it won't work with low- or nonfat mayonnaise.
- For super-crispy fried chicken, use half flour and half cornstarch instead of flour only. Season as usual and add ½ teaspoon baking powder.
- The coating will stick better if you refrigerate the coated chicken, uncovered, for 30 to 60 minutes before cooking.
- Unlike turkeys, chicken, and game hens, you don't want to stuff a duck. The bread in the stuffing absorbs so much fat that it becomes inedible.
- Farm-raised ducks are so fatty that they don't require basting.
- When stuffing a game hen, count on about 1 cup dressing per bird.
- Are you a city slicker in search of wild game? You can order some by mail order. Broken Arrow Ranch carries American venison and many other types of game, like antelope and boar. Call 800-962-4263 and request a catalog.

Chicken Parmesan Florentine

Contributed by Deborah Taylor-Hough

4 Servings

4 boneless and skinless chicken breasts
2 eggs, beaten in small bowl
  dry bread crumbs
4 slices mozzarella cheese
  Parmesan cheese
1 package frozen spinach, cooked and drained
3 cups spaghetti sauce (homemade or good quality from a
  jar)
1 package egg noodles
  butter
  fresh parsley, finely chopped

Cook egg noodles according to package instructions, drain, and return to cooking pan. Drop in about 2 tablespoons butter and stir until noodles are lightly buttered. Sprinkle with 1 teaspoon chopped parsley and keep warm.

Pound chicken breasts until thin and of a consistent thickness (approximately ¼ inch). Dip chicken into beaten egg, then into bread crumbs to coat lightly. Broil chicken breasts until cooked through, turning halfway through cooking time. Place one slice of mozzarella on each chicken breast and sprinkle generously with Parmesan cheese. Put under broiler only until mozzarella melts and Parmesan cheese starts to turn light brown. Layer ingredients onto individual serving dishes in the following order: noodles, spinach, spaghetti sauce and then chicken breasts. Sprinkle lightly with more Parmesan. Serve with hot garlic bread. Enjoy!

Nutrient value per serving: 563 calories, 65 g protein, 24 g fat, 22 g carbohydrates, 1,396 mg sodium, 266 mg cholesterol.

Alternative: For a more traditional chicken Parmesan, prepare any sort of homemade béchamel sauce, cook the chicken breasts in the same fashion as above, including cheeses, and omit the spaghetti sauce and spinach. Set chicken on individual serving plates and spoon white sauce over top. Sprinkle with chopped parsley. Serve beside buttered noodles sprinkled with Parmesan cheese and parsley. This meal is a little bland looking (white-on-white), but if you serve it with a colorful tossed green salad and a broiled tomato crown, it looks a lot better. It's also helpful if you serve it on very vibrant, colorful plates!

Creamy Chicken Enchiladas
Contributed by Nancy Guth
4 Servings

8 corn tortillas
2 cups Jack cheese, grated
6 green onions, chopped
2 10¾ ounces can condensed cream of chicken soup
8 ounces sour cream
1 4 ounce can chopped green chilies
½ teaspoon salt
1 tablespoon oil, for frying
4 chicken breasts, cooked and cubed

In a medium saucepan heat chicken soup, sour cream, chilies, and salt until hot. Add cubed chicken to the sauce. Fry tortillas in a small amount of hot oil for about 5 seconds each until soft. On each tortilla place ¼ cup cheese, some onion, and 2 tablespoons sauce. Roll and place seam-side down in a 2-quart casserole. Pour remaining sauce over the top, covering well. Bake 20 to 30 minutes at 350°.

Nutrient value per serving: 1,059 calories, 82 g protein, 59 g fat, 50 g carbohydrates, 2,507 mg sodium, 243 mg cholesterol.

Crispy Baked Pheasant
Contributed by Jeanne Young
6 Servings

If pheasant is not available, chicken makes a nice substitute.

1   pheasant, cut up, OR 1 whole chicken, cut up
1¼   teaspoons salt, divided
⅓   cup all-purpose flour
¼   teaspoon cayenne pepper
2   tablespoons milk
1   egg, slightly beaten
¾   cup cornflake crumbs, or other crushed cereal
4   tablespoons butter or margarine, melted
3   tablespoons lemon juice

Sprinkle pheasant evenly with 1 teaspoon of salt. In a bowl combine flour, pepper, and remaining salt. In another bowl whisk together the milk and egg. Cereal crumbs require a third bowl. Dredge each piece in flour mixture, egg mixture, and crumbs, pressing crumbs evenly onto the pheasant. Place in an ungreased 13 x 9-inch baking dish. Mix together the butter and lemon juice and drizzle over pheasant. Bake at 375° for 45 minutes or until juices run clear.

Nutrition value per serving with pheasant: 256 calories, 27 g protein, 12 g fat, 10 g carbohydrates, 654 mg sodium, less than 1 g cholesterol.

Holiday Hens with Apricots and Cranberries
4 Servings

1 cup dried apricot halves
1 cup cranberries, dried
4 tablespoons olive oil
2 small onions, finely chopped
4 cloves garlic, finely chopped
4 teaspoons ginger root, grated
1 teaspoon ground cinnamon
1 16 ounce can tomato sauce
2 tablespoons brown sugar, packed
  salt, to taste
  pepper, to taste
  seasoned salt, to taste
4 Cornish game hens

Combine apricots and cranberries in a small bowl. Let stand for one hour. Drain, reserving liquid. Preheat oven to 375°. Heat 1 tablespoon olive oil in medium pan. Add onion, garlic, and ginger root, and sauté for 5 minutes over medium heat. Add reserved liquid, fruit, cinnamon, tomato sauce, and brown sugar. Season with salt and pepper. Simmer for 5 minutes. Pour mixture into a small roasting pan. Rinse hens with cold water and pat dry with paper towels. Discard any obvious fat. Sprinkle hen cavities with seasoned salt and pepper. Rub skins lightly with olive oil. Arrange hens over sauce in pan. Bake until golden, basting occasionally with pan juices, 1 hour to 1 hour and 15 minutes.

Nutrient value per serving: 1,448 calories, 99 g protein, 94 g fat, 43 g carbohydrates, 1,495 mg sodium, 557 mg cholesterol.

Honey-Glazed Pheasant
Contributed by Jeanne Young
6 Servings

If pheasant is not available, chicken makes a nice substitute.

½ cup all-purpose flour
1 teaspoon salt
½ teaspoon cayenne pepper
1 pheasant, cut up, OR 1 whole chicken, cut up
½ cup butter or margarine, melted and divided
¼ cup brown sugar, packed
¼ cup honey
¼ cup lemon juice
2 tablespoons soy sauce

In a bowl combine flour, salt, and pepper; add meat pieces and dredge to coat. Pour 4 tablespoons butter into a 13 x 3 x 9-inch baking dish. Place pheasant pieces in pan, turning to coat. Bake, uncovered, at 350° for 30 minutes. Combine brown sugar, honey, lemon juice, soy sauce, and remaining butter in a saucepan; heat on stove top set at low for 15 to 20 minutes. Pour over pheasant. Bake 45 minutes more or until pheasant is tender, basting several times with pan drippings.

Nutrition value per serving with pheasant: 376 calories, 26 g protein, 19 g fat, 26 g carbohydrates, 923 mg sodium, 26 mg cholesterol.

Parmesan Pheasant
Contributed by Jeanne Young
6 Servings

If pheasant is not available, chicken makes a nice substitute.

1 pheasant, cut up, OR 6 chicken breasts
½ cup butter or margarine, melted
2 teaspoons mustard
1 teaspoon Worcestershire sauce
½ teaspoon salt
1 cup cracker crumbs
½ cup Parmesan cheese, grated

In a bowl combine butter, mustard, Worcestershire sauce, and salt. In another bowl combine crumbs and Parmesan cheese. Dip pheasant in butter mixture, then the crumb mixture. Place in an ungreased 13 x 9-inch baking dish. Drizzle with any remaining butter mixture. Bake at 350°. for 45 minutes or until juices run clear.

Nutrition value per serving with pheasant: 366 calories, 29 g protein, 23 g fat, 11 g carbohydrates, 717 mg sodium, 1g cholesterol.

Russian Apricot Chicken
Contributed by Paulette Hegg
8 Servings

3½ pounds whole chicken, cut up and skinned
    salt and pepper to taste
1 onion, chopped
2 to 3 cloves garlic, chopped
½ pound apricot preserves
6 ounces Russian salad dressing

Preheat oven to 350°. Season the chicken well with salt and pepper and lay in large baking dish. Add chopped onion and garlic. Mix together the apricot preserves and Russian dressing. Pour over the chicken and bake about 50 minutes covered.

Nutrient value per serving: 538 calories, 41 g protein, 31 g fat, 25 g carbohydrates, 307 mg sodium, 25 mg cholesterol.

Southern Fried Chicken
4 Servings

2 cups buttermilk, preferably salt-free
⅛ teaspoon salt
¼ teaspoon black pepper, freshly ground
¼ teaspoon cayenne
10 pieces chicken (2 wings, 2 thighs, 2 legs, 4 breast pieces
     cut in half, OR substitute 2 pounds boneless chicken
     breasts, skin intact)
⅔ cups whole wheat flour
⅔ cup all-purpose flour
1½ teaspoons salt
1 teaspoon black pepper, freshly ground
½ teaspoon cayenne
    Crisco for frying

In a shallow, nonaluminum dish, combine first four ingredients. Add chicken and toss once to coat. Cover and chill 8 hours or overnight, turning once or twice.

Place pieces on rack to drain slightly, but do not pat dry.

In a paper bag combine flours, salt, black pepper, and cayenne. Toss chicken in flour mixture and place on a clean rack or a baking sheet. Toss each piece again, shake off excess flour and set aside until ready to fry.

In 2 large, heavy skillets, or 1 electric skillet, heat enough Crisco oil to reach a depth of ½ inch at 350° to 360° (be sure to test temperature with thermometer). Add chicken pieces to the hot oil one by one. (Note: Adding too many pieces at once lowers the temperature of the oil, and the chicken will not brown properly.) Adjust temperature so oil remains between 300° and 320°. Cook, turning once with tongs, 10 to 12 minutes per side (4 to 5 minutes for boneless breasts) or until juices run clear when pierced in the thickest part. (Thicker pieces may require more cooking time.) As they are done, transfer pieces to paper towels to drain. Serve hot or warm.

Gravy for fried chicken: Drain all the oil from the cooking skillet through a sieve and into a bowl. Return the skillet to medium heat.

Add 2 tablespoons of the chicken-frying fat to the skillet, along with any browned bits caught by the strainer. Add 2 tablespoons of flour, blend well, and cook for 2 minutes, stirring. Remove from heat, add a scant 2 cups boiling chicken stock. Simmer for 2 minutes, season (using freshly grated nutmeg, if desired), and serve.

Nutrient value per serving: 541 calories, 63 g protein, 16 g fat, 37 g carbohydrates, 404 mg sodium, 157 mg cholesterol.

Chapter 12

*P*asta, Grains, and Rice

MUCH MORE THAN MOUNDS OF CARBOHYDRATES

A gourmet meal is one that I can proudly serve to guests
without feeling that I have sacrificed taste
for the sake of cutting costs.
—June Rich

Back a decade or so ago when we found out that carbohydrates were our friends, America embraced all forms of pasta. Up until that time, unless you grew up with Italian neighbors or were of Italian ancestry, an average American's exposure to pasta was spaghetti, and if you were like me, you didn't know that *spaghetti* meant the shape of the pasta, not the sauce. Now that we are so much more educated on the subject, an entire world of Epicurean possibilities has opened up.

Basically pasta is the general name for the variously shaped flour and water dough products, which happen to include many members in its family. Pasta may be white, egg-enriched yellow, or spinach green—although lately you can find pasta in every color of the rainbow, made from every imaginable kind of vegetable, flour, or grain. The real difference in pasta lies not in its shapes, however, but whether it is domestic, imported, or homemade.

American factory-made pasta tends to be too gummy when cooked, and it is often hard to separate the strands. This is caused by the type of flour and used to be the standard for pasta available in the grocery store. However, with the rapidly growing popularity of pasta, American pasta-makers have turned to their Italian counterparts for a more authentic version. You can now buy pretty decent domestic pasta in your local store, as long as you only purchase brands made with durum wheat, also called semolina.

In the past you could only find imported, factory-made dry pasta in the local Italian grocery. You can still get great pasta in Italian groceries and delis, but now many good brands are available in your regular market. If you are interested in fresh pasta and don't want to make it yourself, the Italian grocery is still your best bet. Whether you make your own pasta or buy it fresh, stock up and freeze it. When you cook it, take it directly from the freezer and place in boiling water.

Sauces for pasta dishes have become more adventurous by the minute, although several have stood the test of time and have survived the goat cheese, duck, and spicy pepper trends. They are creamy Alfredo sauce, carbonara sauce, four-cheese sauce, classic tomato sauce, pesto sauce, and seafood sauce. Mastering any or all of these will instantly expand your repertoire with entrées, vegetables, and pastas, not to mention equipping you with the ability to create your own sauces from standard items in the refrigerator or pantry. Because pasta cooks so quickly and making a sauce is a snap, dinner can be ready in no time.

Rice and Grains

There is a reason that rice is the staple food for most of the world's population. It's filling, nutritious, and very tolerant of being turned into a main dish, salad, or side dish. Once American chefs started experimenting with the more unusual and healthy fare, the American consumer realized that rice wasn't just white and grain wasn't just something animals ate.

Nowadays it's very normal for most cooks to regularly serve meals that include white, brown, and wild rice; lentils; couscous; and risotto. And the great thing is that because rice and grains are so filling and good for you, a very elegant yet simple meal can be prepared and served along with nothing more than a salad. And no one realizes there's no meat on the plate!

Without going on about the wonderful aspects of rice and grains, I have to mention how economical they are. Thus, experimenting is rather fun because if your couscous experiment flops, you haven't ruined your food budget for the week. If your family is still a little gun-shy about that strange-looking mound on their plate, there are still great ways to spiff up classic white rice. (When referring to white rice I do *not* mean instant or "minute" rice: I mean long-grain white rice. Some would say that since the creation of minute rice, an eleventh commandment should be added: *"Thou shalt not allow minute rice to pass thy lips."* I might add that they would rather eat cardboard—as it has more flavor and personality.) If you are a fan of minute rice, don't be offended, but you might want to venture out into the long-grain variety. It'll only add about 30 minutes to your time, but it's worth it.

To white rice add grated cheese before cooking; after cooking stir in about two cups of chopped ham, beef, or poultry; or chill and add your favorite salad dressing and chilled cooked vegetables.

Four standard types of rice are the most popular. White rice has its outer covering removed by a process called "polishing." Converted rice is hulled under moist conditions, steamed, and dried so that all the nutrients are incorporated back into the grain; how-ever, it tastes a little pasty. Brown rice is superior to white rice in nutrients because it retains its outer coating. Although it takes longer to cook than white rice, its good, nutty flavor and high food value make it very popular. Finally, wild rice is not rice at all but the seed from a grass that grows wild along the edges of lakes in Michigan, Minnesota, Wisconsin, and southern Canada. It is har-vested by bending the grasses over the side of a boat and beating the seeds into the boats. It is more expensive, dark in color, strong and intriguing in taste, and well worth the occasional indulgence.

A fifth type that is becoming very popular is arborio rice, which is short-grain, high-starch rice that is the basis for risotto. The use of arborio in the preparation of risotto is how it differs from standard white rice. For risotto, hot liquid is added to the rice, about ½ cup at a time, stirring constantly until the rice absorbs the liquid. Once absorbed, the next ½ cup of liquid is added, and so on until all the liquid has cooked down.

Tips

♦ Store white rice in an airtight container in a cool, dark place for up to one year; store brown rice for up to six months. In warm climates, or for longer storage, refrigerate or freeze rice.

♦ A teaspoon or two of lemon juice in the cooking water will make cooked rice whiter.

♦ One or two teaspoons of vegetable oil added to the cooking water will keep it from boiling over.

♦ Adding oil or butter to the water will also keep the grains from sticking together.

♦ If rice is scorched, the best thing to do is start over. However, if that's not an option, place the heel of a loaf of bread on top of the rice, cover the pot, and wait five minutes. Most of the scorched taste should disappear into the bread.

♦ Add leftover rice to soups and stews at the last minute so the rice doesn't get soft and mushy.

♦ For fluffy, cold rice pudding, fold softly whipped cream into chilled rice pudding.

♦ Fresh pasta can be wrapped airtight in a plastic bag and refrigerated for up to five days, or double wrapped and frozen for up to four months.

♦ To skip the step of transferring pasta from the pot to the colander to rinse, cook pasta in a pot with a removable inner basket, or use a metal colander or large strainer inside a pot of boiling water. Lift out and rinse.

♦ Unsalted water will reach a boil faster than salted water, so add salt to rapidly boiling water just before adding the pasta.

♦ If cooked pasta sticks together, spritz it gently with hot running water for just a few seconds. Drain.

♦ Invest in the gadget called a spaghetti fork or spaghetti server. It looks like a weird spoon with claws and makes serving a whole lot easier. You can also use two large forks or tongs.

California Couscous
8 Servings

A fabulous alternative to rice.

1½ cups chicken broth
2 teaspoons curry power
1 cup couscous
2 cloves garlic, minced
½ cup celery, chopped
½ cup onions, chopped
1 tablespoon olive oil
¼ cup chopped chutney
3 tablespoons lemon juice
¼ cup toasted pine nuts
¼ cup dried currants
½ cup green onions including tops, thinly sliced

Boil chicken broth and curry powder in a medium saucepan. Add couscous, stir, cover, and reduce heat to low. Cook for 5 minutes longer. Remove from heat and fluff with a fork. Cover until ready to use.

While couscous cooks, sauté garlic, celery, and onion in oil over medium heat until soft but not browned; about 5 minutes. Combine chutney and lemon juice together in small bowl.

Toss couscous with vegetable mixture. Stir pine nuts, currants, and green onions into chutney mixture. This can be done in a frying pan over low heat. Serve immediately or place in a casserole and briefly reheat at serving time.

Nutrient value per serving: 181 calories, 4 g protein, 5 g fat, 30 g carbohydrates, 289 mg sodium, 0 mg cholesterol.

Fettucine Parmesan
Contributed by Judy Bergman
6 Servings

1   pound bacon, cut into small pieces
1   onion, chopped
4   cloves garlic, diced or pressed
1   pound fresh mushrooms, sliced
¾   liter chicken stock
1   pound fettucine
4   egg whites
6   ounces Parmesan cheese

Sauté bacon until partially done. Remove most of grease and add onions and garlic. Sauté until onions are soft. Add chicken stock and simmer 10 to 15 minutes. Boil fettucine noodles until done. While noodles are cooking (about 5 minutes before they are done), add mushrooms to the bacon mixture. Drain noodles. Stir in beaten eggs to noodles (the heat from the noodles will cook the eggs perfectly). Add Parmesan cheese to noodles; toss well. Add bacon mixture to noodles. Mix and serve.

Nutrient value per serving: 633 calories, 39 g protein, 22 g fat, 52 g carbohydrates, 1,579 mg sodium, 135 mg cholesterol.

Fresh Asparagus Risotto
5 Servings

1 pound fresh asparagus
4 cups chicken stock or vegetable stock
1 stick butter
1 onion, peeled and chopped
1 cup arborio rice, uncooked
2 tablespoons whipping cream
½ cup Parmesan cheese
2 tablespoons butter
  salt and freshly ground white pepper, to taste
  chopped tomato for garnish

Discard tough ends of aparagus. Reserve the tips for later use in the recipe. Thinly slice the trimmed, tender stalks leaving the tips in 1-inch pieces. Bring the stock to a boil in a medium saucepan; reduce heat to a slow simmer. Place a ladle next to the saucepan.

In a large wide saucepan, melt butter over medium-high heat. Add onion and cook, stirring occasionally, until onions are transparent but not browned. Add rice and stir rapidly to coat rice with butter. Add asparagus slices.

Add ¼ to 1 cup stock so that the rice is barely covered with liquid. Stirring frequently, allow stock to evaporate and to be absorbed. Don't allow the rice to go completely dry. Keep adding stock in ¼ cup measurements until 1 cup of stock remains to be added to the rice.

Add the asparagus tips and finish adding stock ½ cup at a time. When all the stock has been absorbed, remove pan from heat. Immediately stir in whipping cream, Parmesan cheese, and butter. Add salt and pepper to taste.

Presentation: Divide among 5 bowls. If desired, garnish with chopped tomato. Serve immediately.

Nutrient value per serving: 335 calories, 11 g protein, 11 g fat, 40 g carbohydrates, 1,408 mg sodium, 28 mg cholesterol.

Italian Lasagna
Best lasagna in the free world!
12 Servings

1   pound lasagna noodles
1   onion, diced
2   cloves garlic, chopped
1   tablespoon oil
2   cups tomato paste, and 2 cups water
2   cups fresh mushrooms, sliced, OR 2 cans mushrooms, drained
2   12 ounce cans tomato purée, plus 2 cans of water
½   teaspoon basil
½   teaspoon oregano
1   tablespoon sugar
1   teaspoon salt
½   teaspoon Italian herb seasoning
3   pounds ground beef, top round
1   pound Italian sausage, with fennel
2   pounds mozzarella cheese, sliced
2   pounds ricotta cheese
4   eggs, slightly beaten
¼   cup romano cheese, or Parmesan cheese, grated

Brown onions and garlic in oil; add purée, paste, water, mushrooms, herbs, and seasonings. Brown meat and sausage, drain fat, and add meat to sauce. Simmer 2 to 3 hours. Cook noodles in boiling water for 8 minutes. Drain, rinse, and lay out flat. Gently stir beaten eggs into ricotta cheese. Fill a large lasagna pan in layers as follows: sauce, lasagna noodles, sauce, mozzarella, ricotta. Repeat these layers until all ingredients are in the pan. Bake in 350° oven for 20 to 30 minutes or until mozzarella is melted.

Nutrient value per serving: 935 calories, 67 g protein, 53 g fat, 49 g carbohydrates, 1,126 mg sodium, 285 mg cholesterol.

Lasagna Swirls
8 Servings

8 lasagna noodles
1 10 ounce package frozen chopped spinach, thawed
   and drained
1 cup Parmesan cheese
1⅓ cups ricotta cheese
½ teaspoon salt
¼ teaspoon pepper
¼ teaspoon nutmeg

Sauce:
4 cloves garlic, minced
2 onions, large
4 tablespoons oil
2 15 ounce can tomato sauce
2 teaspoons sugar
1 teaspoon salt
½ teaspoon pepper
1 teaspoon basil, crumbled
1 teaspoon oregano, crumbled

Mix together the spinach, ¾ cup of the Parmesan cheese, ricotta, salt, pepper, and nutmeg while the noodles are cooking. When they are al dente and cool enough to handle, spread about ⅓ cup of the cheese mixture along the entire length of each noodle. Roll the noodles and stand on end in a greased 8-inch round casserole that is at least two and one half inches deep.

Sauté garlic and onion in the oil over medium heat. When limp, add the tomato sauce, sugar, salt, pepper, basil, and oregano. Simmer uncovered for five minutes. Pour over the noodles, cover, and bake at 350° for about 30 minutes or until the casserole is thoroughly hot. This will be about an hour if it has been refrigerated. Remove from the oven and sprinkle with the remaining ¼ cup Parmesan cheese.

Nutrient value per serving: 207 calories, 12 g protein, 13 g fat, 11 g carbohydrates, 907 mg sodium, 31 mg cholesterol.

Manicotti Stuffed with Zucchini and Tofu
Contributed by Paulette Hegg
6 Servings

This is one of my favorite recipes. No one will ever know it has tofu in it if you don't tell them. It tastes like cheese.

2	teaspoons olive oil
½	onion, finely chopped
¼	teaspoon marjoram
¼	teaspoon basil
3	cloves garlic, chopped
¼	green bell pepper, finely chopped
6	mushrooms, chopped
2	small zucchinis, or 1 large, chopped
2	tablespoons parsley
1½	cups tomatoes, chopped
¼	teaspoon pepper
¼	teaspoon paprika
	dash of salt
1	pound firm tofu, drained and crumbled
½	teaspoon honey
½	teaspoon salt
	dash nutmeg
2	teaspoons lemon juice
12 to 14	manicotti shells, cooked
	tomato sauce

In large skillet, heat oil. Add onion, marjoram, and basil. Cover and cook until onion is tender. Add chopped garlic and cook 1 minute. Chop green pepper, mushrooms, and zucchini in food processor or chop by hand. Add to sautéed onion; toss well and cook covered for 5 minutes. Add parsley, tomatoes, pepper, paprika, and dash of salt and cook covered for 10 minutes. Remove cover and cook another 5 minutes. There should be no liquid in bottom of pan.

Meanwhile in a blender combine tofu, honey, ½ teaspoon salt, nutmeg, and lemon juice and blend until smooth. Stir into the vegetables.

Turn oven to 350°. Gently fill each cooked manicotti shell with above mixture. Lightly cover the bottom of a large baking dish with tomato sauce. Set manicotti shells side by side in dish and cover with more tomato sauce. Bake, covered, for 20 minutes. Remove cover and bake 15 minutes more.

Nutrient value per serving: 179 calories, 14 g protein, 9 g fat, 11 g carbohydrates, 409 mg sodium, 0 mg cholesterol.

Pasta Salad
Contributed by Judy Bergman

I purposely did not include amounts because this recipe can be made for an army or for two. Feel free to substitute ingredients for what's fresh and in season. The most important ingredient is the salad dressing. It must be Bernstein's. As far as I am concerned, no other will do.

tricolor spiral pasta
fresh pressed garlic
green olives, black, or both
fresh tomatoes
red onion, minced
red pepper
green bell pepper
broccoli flowerettes
blue cheese, crumbled
cucumber, diced
sliced salami or pepperoni (optional)
fresh cilantro
Bernstein's Italian Dressing
fresh-grated Parmesan cheese
salt and pepper to taste

Cook the pasta until al dente, drain, and rinse. Rub fresh garlic into the pasta while still warm (about 2 cloves per pound of pasta). Allow to completely cool. Chop remaining ingredients into bite-size pieces. Add dressing to taste. Sprinkle on Parmesan cheese, salt, and pepper. Chill.

Risotto
Contributed by Jan Sandberg
6 Servings

1 small onion, diced
1 chicken giblet, cooked and diced
¼ pound ground round
1 6 ounce jar mushrooms, sliced or stems and pieces
1 tablespoon olive oil
1 tablespoon butter
½ 4 ounce can tomato paste
   juice from mushrooms
1 16 ounce package arborio rice or long-grain rice
   saffron threads, to flavor
   chicken broth to cover

Brown the onion, giblet, ground round, and mushrooms in olive oil and butter. Add the tomato paste, juice, arborio rice, saffron, and enough chicken broth to cover. Cook uncovered for 45 minutes over medium heat, constantly stirring and adding broth to keep covered. Broth will cook down.

Nutrient value per serving: 378 calories, 12 g protein, 8 g fat, 65 g carbohydrates, 44 mg sodium, 46 mg cholesterol.

Risotto with Fennel and Peas
5 Servings

This makes an excellent main dish when accompanied by a salad and bread. Note: Fennel is often labeled "anise" in the supermarkets. It has pale green celery-like stems and bright green, feathery foliage. Trim off the bottom of the stalks and the tough upper stalks above the bulb. Reserve some feathery foliage for a garnish.

6	cups chicken stock or vegetable stock
2	teaspoons olive oil
1	onion, peeled and chopped
1	bunch fresh fennel, trimmed and roughly chopped
1½	cups arborio rice, uncooked
1	cup Parmesan cheese, grated
¾	cup frozen peas, thawed

Place broth in a saucepan and bring to boil; reduce heat to a low simmer.

In a large wide saucepan, heat olive oil on medium-high heat. Add onion and fennel; cook, stirring frequently, until onion is transparent and fennel has softened but not browned. Add rice and stir rapidly to coat rice with oil. Add ⅓ cup of broth and cook, stirring frequently, until most of the liquid has evaporated and been absorbed. Continue adding broth, ½ cup at a time, allowing the liquid to evaporate and be absorbed between additions and stirring frequently. Remove from heat, add cheese, and vigorously stir until blended. Gently stir in peas.

Presentation: Divide among 5 bowls. If desired, garnish with sprig of feathery fennel tops. Serve immediately.

Nutrient value per serving: 423 calories, 16 g protein, 10 g fat, 58 g carbohydrates, 2,172 mg sodium, 16 mg cholesterol.

Spaghetti Carbonara
8 Servings

4 egg yolks
½ cup heavy cream
⅓ cup Parmesan cheese, grated
¼ cup parsley, chopped
¼ teaspoon salt
¼ teaspoon pepper
1 16 ounce package spaghetti
1 pound bacon, chopped
1 clove garlic, large, or 2 small, minced
3 tablespoons butter

Mix egg yolks, cream, cheese, parsley, salt, and pepper until well blended; set aside. Cook spaghetti according to package directions. Cook bacon pieces and garlic until bacon is well cooked. Pour off about a third of grease. Add to spaghetti and butter; toss well to coat. Add egg mixture; toss and serve.

Nutrient value per serving: 461 calories, 17 g protein, 24 g fat, 44 g carbohydrates, 527 mg sodium, 155 mg cholesterol.

Chapter 13

*V*egetables and Salads

IF THIS IS VEGETABLE, DON'T WAKE ME

*A gourmet meal is one that is presented well, includes
nutritional needs, and is cooked to perfection.*
—Marilyn McCormick

I realize that what I'm about to say might seem a little odd, but one of the most creative areas of cooking is vegetables and salads. No, your mother did not ask me to write that. Just think about it for a minute. In almost every other area of cooking, exact measuring, complementary ingredients, and precise times are required to produce the desired results. But with vegetables your imagination and taste buds are your guide. In the creation and preparation of vegetable dishes and salads, you can experiment and make things up as you go along.

The popularity of vegetables has also contributed to a new attitude: Nowadays, it's cool to like your veggies. You have to wonder why things changed. Was a generation of babies born with some new vegetable-friendly gene? We can only hope, but that's not the reason. There are two, really.

First, it was not so long ago that if you lived on or near a farm, you had access to fresh vegetables. If you didn't, they were more costly and less available. But with this century's dramatic improvements in transportation, cross-country shipments of fresh produce are not only expected but demanded.

Second, attitudes toward vegetable cooking have changed tremendously over the years. Today's emphasis is on preserving the natural goodness of vegetables, cooking them for the shortest possible period of time without leaving them raw. Anyone who grew up on overcooked vegetables, either fresh or canned, learned at an early age to hate them. However, vegetables are finally getting the attention they deserve, especially considering how critical they are to good health.

There are three very important steps involved before your vegetable winds up on your plate or in your salad bowl. Obviously the end result is important, but if buying the freshest and best quality ingredients is important in your other dishes, it's especially true of vegetables. Remember, when served fresh, there's no hiding droopy, wilted salad greens. It obviously depends on what part of the country you live in, but in most areas you can get decent produce in grocery stores or fresh-picked from roadside stands. Produce co-ops are also worth investigating.

In France and other European countries, many people shop for food on a daily basis, with the freshest breads, meats, produce, and dairy products always available. If you shopped like that and consumed most of what you bought, storage wouldn't be such a big deal. But here in America, with our habit of shopping once a week or so, storage of fresh produce is very important. Except for vegetables that need time to ripen, produce should always be stored in the refrigerator until you plan to serve it, ideally within three days.

Don't despair, though, if you had planned to serve those carrots or broccoli tonight, and suddenly your plans changed. Get out of the habit of tossing suspicious vegetables, and cook them before they start to droop, even if you're not going to eat them. Do you know what you can do with them? (No, don't serve steamed broccoli for breakfast!) Freeze them! That's right; any vegetable can be purchased, prepared, and frozen in muffin tins. Allow to freeze slightly, remove, and place in individual freezer containers for later use. This works well for onions, carrots, bell peppers, broccoli, corn (really, anything that you can buy already frozen).

Salad greens (like lettuce) can't be frozen. Unfortunately, their life span is short. But there are things you can do to prolong it a little, or avoid killing it prematurely, mainly through washing, drying, and storing. Wash greens that are dirty as soon as you get them home, using very cold water. (Some of the more compact types of lettuce like iceberg and endive don't need to be washed.) Also, never separate the leaves until you are ready to use them. Avoid wrapping washed greens in plastic bags; they create too much moisture, turning the greens dank more quickly. It's a good idea to check and remove any leaves that have turned brown because they can infect the whole lot. If you have a few leaves that have not gone bad and are crisp enough to serve, use them to line your salad bowl or vegetable platter. This creates a nice touch and puts to good use something that is not edible.

If you are planning to cook your vegetables, most of them can and should be steamed. This gives you the cooked flavor of the vegetable, without that boiled taste, feel, and look. You still have to keep an eye on the time during steaming, as the steam can cook them to a soggy mess, but it's safer than boiling. Both steaming and cooking vegetables in the microwave keep more of the vegetables' nutrients and vitamins intact. Most cooks don't use microwaves for much more than reheating and defrosting, but let me tell you that a microwave cooks a mean vegetable.

The best tip I can give you about vegetables is to explore and experiment. Don't fall for buying the new "designer" vegetables; they may look prettier, but normal veggies can be just as good if their quality is good. Above all, get out of the mind-set that veggies and salads are side dishes. They are basic cheap food and, with some cleverly added ingredients, can turn a standard dish into something memorable.

Tips

♦ The smaller the vegetable, the younger it is and the more tender it will be.

♦ Some vegetables, such as bell peppers and cucumbers, are coated with wax before they're shipped to your store. Waxing is done to extend shelf life, seal in moisture, and improve appearance. The waxes are safe to eat but may contain pesticide residue, so wash carefully all waxed vegetables and fruit.

♦ If you buy root vegetables like beets and carrots with their leaves attached, remove them as soon as you get home (or ask the clerk to remove them). These greens leach the moisture from the vegetable.

♦ Limp vegetables like carrots and potatoes regain much of their crisp texture if soaked in ice water for at least one hour.

♦ Keep blanched vegetables bright and crisp by draining off the hot water, then immediately turning them into a bowl of ice water. Let stand in water only until cool, then drain.

♦ Add ½ to 1 teaspoon sugar to cooked vegetables such as carrots, corn, and peas. This reduces the starchy flavors and highlights natural sweetness.

♦ Make mashed potatoes ahead of time by spooning prepared whipped potatoes into a buttered casserole dish. Dot with pats of butter and cover with plastic wrap and refrigerate. Bake in 350° oven for about 25 minutes or until a knife inserted in the center comes out hot. Or cook in microwave until hot.

♦ Add a good quality mayonnaise along with the butter, salt, and pepper to your cooked potatoes. Prepare as you would for whipped potatoes. Yummy!

♦ While sautéing onions, sprinkle with a bit of sugar if you notice they are browning unevenly. They should begin to cook evenly thereafter.

♦ Boiled onions that have become too soft can be firmed up again by dipping them briefly in ice water.

♦ Cut off a leg of an old clean pair of pantyhose, drop potatoes or onions into it, and hang in a cool, dark, dry place. The hose lets air circulate, which helps keep the onions and potatoes longer. However, because of the interaction of their natural gases, storing potatoes and onions together can cause the potatoes to rot more quickly.

♦ A teaspoon or two of lemon juice in the cooking water will keep potatoes white after cooking.

Artichoke and Rice Salad
6 Servings

1 package rice vermicelli, OR 7 ounce package Rice-A-Roni
   mix; discard seasoning packet
4 green onions, sliced
½ green bell pepper, chopped
12 green olives, stuffed with pimento, sliced
1 5 ounce can water chestnuts, halved
1 6 ounce jar marinated artichoke hearts

Dressing:
⅓ cup mayonnaise
½ teaspoon curry powder

Cook rice mixture according to package directions, omitting the butter. Cool in a large bowl. Add onions, green pepper, olives, and water chestnuts. Drain artichoke hearts, reserving marinade, and cut into bite-sized pieces. Add to rice mixture together with dressing and mix well. Refrigerate overnight for best flavor.

Dressing: Combine mayonnaise and curry powder. Mix well and add the reserved artichoke marinade as necessary to reach the desired consistency.

Nutrient value per serving: 154 calories, 1 g protein, 14 g fat, 6 g carbohydrates, 342 mg sodium, 4 mg cholesterol.

Au Gratin Potatoes
6 Servings

2 pounds potatoes, about 6 medium, washed and peeled
1 onion, medium size, chopped
¼ cup butter
1 tablespoon flour
1 teaspoon salt
¼ teaspoon pepper
2 cups milk
2 cups sharp cheddar cheese, shredded
¼ cup bread crumbs
   paprika

Cut potatoes into enough thin slices to measure about 4 cups. Cook and stir onion in butter in 2-quart saucepan until onion is tender. Stir in flour, salt, and pepper. Cook over low heat, stirring constantly, until mixture is bubbly; remove from heat. Stir in milk and 1½ cups of the cheese. Heat to boiling, stirring constantly. Boil and stir 1 minute. Place potatoes in ungreased 1½-quart casserole. Pour cheese sauce on potatoes. Cook uncovered in 325° oven for 1 hour and 20 minutes or in 375° oven for 1 hour.

Mix remaining cheese and the bread crumbs; sprinkle over potatoes. Sprinkle with paprika. Cook uncovered until top is brown and bubbly, 15 to 20 minutes longer.

Nutrient value per serving: 469 calories, 17 g protein, 23 g fat, 48 g carbohydrates, 782 mg sodium, 71 mg cholesterol.

Broccoli Onion Zucchini Medley
6 Servings

1   pound broccoli, cut into 1½-inch pieces
6   pearl onions, halved
3   zucchini, sliced
1   pound mushrooms, sliced
5   tablespoons butter
3   tablespoons flour
1   cup milk
1   3 ounce package cream cheese, cubed
¼   teaspoon salt
⅛   teaspoon white pepper
½   cup shredded sharp cheddar cheese
1   cup soft bread crumbs

Steam broccoli, onions, zucchini, and mushrooms until al dente. Drain. Melt 3 tablespoons butter over low heat. Add flour and stir until smooth. Gradually add milk and stir until thickened. Remove from heat and add cream cheese. Stir until melted. Add salt and pepper. Add vegetables. Stir gently and spoon into lightly greased 1½-quart casserole dish. Top with cheddar cheese. Cover and bake at 350° for 25 minutes. Melt remaining 2 tablespoons butter and add bread crumbs. Uncover casserole and sprinkle with bread crumbs. Bake uncovered an additional 5 minutes or until golden brown.

Nutrient value per serving: 345 calories, 12 g protein, 21 g fat, 28 g carbohydrates, 464 mg sodium, 58 mg cholesterol.

Chinese Chicken Salad
8 Servings

¼ cup peanut oil
2 tablespoons oriental sesame oil
1 clove garlic, peeled and blanched
1 tablespoon sugar
3 tablespoons rice vinegar
2 tablespoons soy sauce
¼ cup peanut butter
2 tablespoons sesame paste or sesame seeds
   salt and freshly ground pepper
1 teaspoon chili paste with soybeans, optional
2 cups chicken breasts, poached and torn into bite-sized
   pieces
2 cups cooked elbow macaroni
1 10 ounce package frozen petite peas, thawed
2 scallion tops, thinly sliced
   chopped cilantro, optional

In a food processor or blender, combine and purée the peanut and sesame oils, garlic, sugar, rice vinegar, soy sauce, peanut butter, and sesame paste (if using sesame seeds, do not add now). Season to taste with salt and pepper. If desired, stir in chili paste. Pour into large salad bowl. Stir in chicken pieces, macaroni, peas, scallions, and cilantro (and sesame seeds if selected) and mix until well coated. Refrigerate or serve immediately.

Nutrient value per serving: 353 calories, 16 g protein, 3 g fat, 29 g carbohydrates, 321 mg sodium, 24 mg cholesterol.

Curry Chicken Salad
Contributed by Nancy Guth
6 Servings

3 apples
1 cup seedless grapes
½ cup celery, diced small
1½ chicken breasts, cooked and cut into small pieces
¼ cup nuts, chopped

Dressing:
½ cup mayonnaise
1 tablespoon lemon juice
1½ teaspoons curry powder

Core and chop unpeeled apples into small pieces (you need 2 cups of diced apples). Cut grapes in half. Toss apples, grapes, celery, diced chicken, and nuts in a large salad bowl.

Dressing: Combine mayonnaise, lemon juice, and curry powder. Mix well, pour over salad, and toss well. Serve immediately.

Fried Green Tomatoes
4 Servings

1 cup cornmeal
½ cup flour
1 tablespoon sugar
2 pounds green tomatoes, 4 or 5, sliced ½ inch thick
   vegetable oil
   salt and pepper to taste

In a shallow bowl, mix together cornmeal, flour, and sugar.

Dredge both sides of tomatoes in mixture. Press slices firmly into meal so it will make a good coating.

Put enough oil in an iron skillet to come to the depth of about ¼ inch and heat over medium-high heat. Add tomatoes to hot oil a few at a time without crowding, and fry about 2 minutes or until golden brown. Turn and cook other side.

When both sides are golden brown, remove from skillet, drain on paper towels, and sprinkle with salt and pepper to taste. Serve hot.

Nutrient value per serving. 284 calories, 7 g protein, 5 g fat, 53 g carbohydrates, 322 mg sodium, 0 mg cholesterol.

Fumi Salad

Contributed by Lori Hubert

10 Servings

1 head cabbage, chopped
8 tablespoons slivered almonds
8 teaspoons sesame seeds
8 green onion tops, chopped
2 packages Top Ramen noodles, discard seasoning packet
1 tablespoon butter

Dressing:

4 tablespoons sugar
1 teaspoon pepper
1 cup oil
2 teaspoons salt
6 tablespoons rice vinegar

In sauté pan, brown butter, almonds, and sesame seeds. Toss briefly and remove from stove. Allow mixture to cool. In a large salad bowl break raw noodles into pieces, add green onions, chopped cabbage, almonds, and sesame seeds.

Dressing: Combine sugar, pepper, oil, salt, and vinegar in a small jar or bowl. Pour over salad. Toss well and allow to sit for 1 hour before serving.

Nutrient value per serving: 333 calories, 4 g protein, 28 g fat, 15 g carbohydrates, 502 mg sodium, 3 mg cholesterol.

Garlic Dressing
Contributed by Nancy Guth

You're going to love this dressing for many reasons, not the least of which is that you can make it for less than 10 cents a serving! This is a basic, all-purpose salad dressing that's nice to have on hand in a sealed jar, stored in the refrigerator.

1½	cups salad oil
½	cup vinegar
1½	teaspoons salt
1¼	teaspoons sugar
½	teaspoon dry mustard
4	cloves garlic, halved
½	teaspoon tarragon

Mix all ingredients well and pour into a sealable jar. Let stand in sealed jar or other appropriate container overnight before using. Store in refrigerator.

Yield: 2 cups.

Glazed Carrots
Contributed by Paulette Hegg
6 Servings

1½	pounds carrots
1½	tablespoons butter
½	teaspoon ground ginger
2	teaspoons grated orange rind
1	tablespoon honey
1	teaspoon salt

Peel carrots, then slice thin. Place in large saucepan and add remaining ingredients. Cover just barely with water, then bring to a boil. Simmer uncovered until the water has evaporated, about 1 hour. Place in serving bowl; sprinkle with crushed, dried mint; and serve.

Nutrient value per serving: 92 calories, 1 g protein, 3 g fat, 15 g carbohydrates, 457 mg sodium, 8 mg cholesterol.

Grandma Guth's Famous Dressing
Contributed by Ray Guth

1 cup white vinegar
1 cup vegetable oil
1 cup sugar or to taste
1 teaspoon paprika
1 teaspoon salt
1 teaspoon dry mustard
1 teaspoon commercial salad seasoning such as Schilling
    Salad Supreme

Mix well and store in covered container in the refrigerator.
Yield: 2 cups.

Hearts of Palm and Shrimp Salad
6 Servings

¼ cup olive oil
⅛ cup water
1½ teaspoons granulated sugar
1 teaspoon lemon juice
½ teaspoon Dijon mustard
½ teaspoon Worcestershire sauce
½ teaspoon garlic salt
⅛ teaspoon black pepper, ground
2 14 ounce cans hearts of palm, drained
1 pound large shrimp, cooked, peeled, and deveined, OR
    2 cans baby shrimp, rinsed and drained
3 slices bacon, cooked, drained, and crumbled
    red cabbage leaves
    fresh parsley, to garnish

Place oil, vinegar, water, sugar, lemon juice, mustard, Worcestershire
sauce, garlic salt, and pepper in a small bowl and whisk together
until well blended. Cut the hearts of palm in half, lengthwise. Put the
hearts of palm, shrimp, and bacon in a one-gallon resealable bag;
pour in dressing. Seal bag and refrigerate 8 hours or overnight to

allow flavors to blend. Reserve dressing. To serve, artistically arrange the hearts of palm and shrimp on cabbage leaves on individual serving plates. Pour reserved dressing over each salad. Garnish with parsley.

Nutrient value per serving: 277 calories, 23 g protein, 14 g fat, 15 g carbohydrates, 419 mg sodium, 151 mg cholesterol.

Marinated Vegetables
14 Servings

2 16 ounce cans green beans, French style
1 12 ounce can white corn, niblets
1 16 ounce can petite peas
1 cup celery, chopped
1 4 ounce jar pimientoes
¼ cup green onions including tops, minced
1 cup red pepper, diced

Marinating dressing:
¾ cup white vinegar
1 cup sugar
½ cup vegetable oil
1 teaspoon celery seeds

Drain the canned vegetables well. Combine with the fresh ones. In a small saucepan combine marinating ingredients and heat, stirring, until sugar is dissolved. Cool slightly and pour over vegetables and allow to marinate overnight.

Nutrient value per serving: 207 calories, 4 g protein, 8 g fat, 29 g carbohydrates, 88 mg sodium, 0 mg cholesterol.

Mediterranean Salad Dressing

1 cup olive oil
2 tablespoons feta cheese, crumbled
1 teaspoon Dijon mustard
2 cloves garlic, minced
4 to 8 anchovies
1 teaspoon Worcestershire sauce
½ cup Parmesan cheese, grated
    lemon juice
    salt and pepper to taste

Combine all ingredients in food processor fitted with metal blade.
Process. Makes a thick Caesar-style dressing.
Yield: 1½ cups.
Use over hearts of romaine lettuce or as a dip for crusty bread.

Paradise Salad
6 Servings

Candied Almonds:
½ cup sliced almonds
3 tablespoons sugar

Salad:
½ head green leaf lettuce, torn into bite-size pieces
½ head romaine lettuce, torn into bite-size pieces
1 cup chopped celery
4 green onions, chopped
1 10¾ ounce can mandarin orange sections, drained
1 avocado, cut into chunks
1 apple, diced
¼ cup dried currants
½ cup bleu cheese, crumbled
3 chicken breast halves, cooked and shredded

Dressing:
½ teaspoon salt

½ teaspoon pepper
¼ cup oil
1 tablespoon chopped parsley
2 tablespoons sugar

Candied almonds: Melt 3 tablespoons sugar in large frying pan with sliced almonds, stirring continuously until almonds are coated. Caution: Don't allow sugar to caramelize. Spread out on wax paper to cool. Mix together all salad ingredients and candied almonds.

   Dressing: Combine salt, pepper, oil, parsley, and sugar; pour over salad and toss right before serving.

   Nutrient value per serving: 492 calories, 20 g protein, 27 g fat, 42 g carbohydrates, 388 mg sodium, 47 mg cholesterol.

   Recommendation: Make an additional batch of dressing to pass with salad.

Petite Pea Salad
8 Servings

1   16 ounce package frozen petite peas
10 slices bacon
¼   cup red onions, finely diced
½   cup celery, finely diced
¼   cup almonds, finely chopped

Dressing:

1   cup sour cream
½   cup mayonnaise
2   tablespoons lemon juice
1   teaspoon sugar

Place frozen peas in a colander. Rinse with cool water and allow to drain while defrosting. Sauté bacon until well done. Allow to cool and crumble into tiny pieces. Combine thawed peas, crumbled bacon, diced onion, and diced celery in a large salad bowl.

   Dressing: Mix sour cream, mayonnaise, lemon juice, and sugar in a small container or bowl. Fold dressing into salad. Add nuts and stir briefly.

Nutrient value per serving: 301 calories, 8 g protein, 25 g fat, 12 g carbohydrates, 324 mg sodium, 25 mg cholesterol.

Prosciutto Wrapped Asparagus
Contributed by Margaret Gamble
25 Servings

3 pounds fresh asparagus, about 50 spears
   Dijon mustard
1 pound prosciutto, or smoked ham, thinly sliced

Trim tough ends off asparagus and remove scales from stalks with a knife or vegetable peeler. Cook asparagus in a small amount of boiling water 3 or 4 minutes. Plunge asparagus into ice water. Drain. Spread about ⅛ teaspoon mustard on one side of each slice of prosciutto or ham. Wrap mustard side around asparagus. Cover and chill up to 2 days.

Nutrient value per serving: 41 calories, 6 g protein, 1 g fat, 2 g carbohydrates, 238 mg sodium, 5 mg cholesterol.

Provençal Feast
Contributed by Betty Coates
8 Servings

This dish can be easily expanded by adding additional vegetables such as blanched green beans, small boiled red potatoes, red onion slices (dipped in the olive oil and baked with the eggplant), grilled chicken tenderloins, and black olives.

3 Japanese eggplants
   olive oil
   salt and pepper to taste
3 cloves garlic, minced
1 long French or Italian baguette cut into thin diagonal slices
   aioli (see below)
   assorted baby lettuces mixed with fresh basil leaves
2 to 3 vine-ripened tomatoes

  1   tablespoon balsamic vinegar
  ½   pound fontina cheese, sliced
       optional garnish: assorted fresh herbs

Aioli sauce:
  3   cloves garlic, peeled
  ⅓   cup red bell peppers
  1   cup mayonnaise
  1   pinch cayenne

Cut eggplants into ½-inch slices on the diagonal. Place in a bowl with olive oil to lightly coat the slices; season with salt and pepper. Place in a single layer in jelly-roll pan and sprinkle with minced garlic. Bake for 20 minutes in a preheated 350° oven. Cool.

Presentation: Place bowl of aioli sauce in the center of a large platter. Arrange vegetables, cheese, chicken, and bread on a bed of baby lettuces and basil surrounding the bowl. Sprinkle tomatoes with balsamic vinegar or seasoned salt. Guests serve themselves with individual plates or make portable treats by assembling small sandwiches.

Sauce: Mince garlic in food processor or blender. Blend in red pepper. Blend in mayonnaise and cayenne. Process until smooth. Refrigerate in airtight container.

Side Bar
Contributed by Julie Harper
4 Servings

I want to share a wonderful basic recipe I've used over and over. Since I've never known the official name of this recipe, I named it Side Bar because my husband is an attorney. This dish is good with chicken, beef, pork, or an all-vegetable menu.

1   10 ounce package frozen spinach
1½   ounces cream cheese
½   stick butter
3   tablespoons Parmesan cheese
1   pinch salt

Cook the spinach according to package directions. Drain excess liquid or squeeze off water. Put cooked spinach in an ovenproof dish. Melt cream cheese and butter over low heat. Add to spinach. Add salt. Stir. Top with Parmesan cheese. Bake in oven at 375° until heated through. Note: Cream cheese and Parmesan cheese may be increased or decreased according to personal taste.

Nutrient value per serving: 93 calories, 5 g protein, 7 g fat, 3 g carbohydrates, 767 mg sodium, 19 mg cholesterol.

Spinach Dip
12 Servings

1   loaf French bread, unsliced
1   package Knorr dry vegetable soup mix
1   cup mayonnaise
1   cup sour cream
1   10 ounce package frozen spinach, thawed and completely
      drained
1   6 ounce can water chestnuts, finely chopped
½   onion, finely chopped

Mix all ingredients (except bread) together, blending well. Refrigerate for at least two hours or overnight. In the meantime cut "top" off loaf of French bread. Lay the lid aside and carefully scoop out bread from inside, creating a "boat" or "basket." Fill cavity with dip mixture. Cover with "lid" until ready to serve. Serve with chips, crackers, and bread pieces for dipping.

Nutrient value per serving: 357 calories, 5 g protein, 20 g fat, 25 g carbohydrates, 354 mg sodium, 15 mg cholesterol.

Succulent Creamed Corn
8 Servings

1½   cups half-and-half
 2   cubes chicken bouillon
 1   dash white pepper
 2   teaspoons sugar
 2   10 ounce packages frozen corn, thawed
 2   tablespoons butter
 2   tablespoons flour
     fresh parsley, chopped

Blend together half-and-half, chicken bouillon cubes, pepper, and sugar in saucepan. Bring to boil. Add corn to boiling liquid. Return to boil, reduce heat, and simmer 3 to 5 minutes. Melt butter in separate small saucepan. Add flour and cook, stirring constantly, until paste is formed. Add flour mixture to corn mixture and stir with wooden spoon to mix well. Bring to boil, stirring frequently, until thickened. Remove from heat. Sprinkle lightly with chopped parsley.

Nutrient value per serving: 163 calories, 4 g protein, 9 g fat, 18 g carbohydrates, 329 mg sodium, 25 mg cholesterol.

Sweet Potato Latkes
Contributed by Paulette Hegg
6 Servings

A favorite dish for Hanukkah.

2   pounds peeled sweet potatoes
1   onion
2   large eggs
¾   teaspoon salt
¼   teaspoon pepper
5   tablespoons flour
    oil

Grate the potatoes and onion by hand or in food processor. Mix all the ingredients. Heat oil in sauté pan until just before it begins to smoke. Using a large tablespoon or round spatula, spoon a round portion of the mixture into the hot oil and brown slightly on both sides. Serve hot with sour cream or applesauce. This will serve 4 to 6 depending on how many you eat before they leave the kitchen.

Nutrient value per serving: 243 calories, 6 g protein, 4 g fat, 45 g carbohydrates, 333 mg sodium, 71 mg cholesterol.

Chapter 14

$\mathscr{P}$astries and Desserts

THE PIÈCE DE RÉSISTANCE!

*A gourmet meal . . . quietly affirms a smooth balance of
flavor, texture, and appearance. Above all, it tastes great
twice—at the table
and thereafter in the memory!*
—Barbara Nosek

I have not met a person yet who does not like at least a little something after dinner. Even if it's just a few fresh berries with a dollop of cream, dessert adds closure to a meal, rounds it out, sends a signal to the palate that "all is well, you did a good job, time to rest."

Now the type of dessert is the real order of business here. First let me say that you must have a real passion for dessert—to eat it, create it, and prepare it—to be a great dessert gourmet. That's not to say that if you're ambivalent about dessert your only options are either to ignore it entirely or hit the gourmet bakery. What I am saying is to choose your struggles wisely. Don't enter into battle with a croquembouche if your only area of expertise is being able to bake a mean Pillsbury slice-and-bake refrigerator cookie. There are many ways to turn ordinary box cakes, ice cream, or fresh fruit into elegant desserts.

If desserts and pastries aren't your thing and you have no desire to change, don't! The secret to a real gourmet cook, especially one just starting out, is to pick your area of interest and stick with it.

Now, for those of you who would just as soon skip the entire process of dinner and fast forward to dessert, I'm with you. There is nothing so elegant and impressive as a grand and glorious creation of sweets. Here's the key to the whole thing, though—your dessert and dinner must be in perfect balance. A heavy dessert after a heavy meal is disaster. Remember that after you've put your heart and soul into preparing a dessert, you want your guests to enjoy it, appreciate it, be blown away by it! So the time for your triple-layer double-fudge torte is not after a heavy meal of lasagna, bread, and salad. You present this creation after that type of a meal, and two things will happen: Most guests will pass and skip to the coffee, and those partaking will never truly enjoy the significance of this final course.

So what do you do? It's simple. Decide ahead of time whether you're going to plan your meal around the entrée or the dessert. It's that easy. A light meal enhances an "out of this world" dessert, and a simple dessert rounds out a dinner that was to die for.

In this chapter we will cover a range of skills and interests in preparing a dessert, and the recipes at the end reflect this range. I have also included ideas and recipes for making and serving gourmet coffees and creamers, which are a natural accompaniment to dessert.

When planning a dessert, you can do everything from scratch or borrow from store-bought prepared foods that you might stock in your pantry. A simple idea can very often turn out to be the most impressive. For example, a sprinkling of a favorite flavored syrup gives a sophisticated taste to store-bought ice cream that has been spread between layers of store-bought cake (or a cake you prepared from a box mix). When you decorate it with whipped cream and chopped nuts and serve it with a fruit sauce, it looks and tastes like a million.

For the purist, box cake mixes are a turnoff, but for those of us with not a lot of time or interest, it can be the beginning of a really great dessert. Prepare and bake the cake according to package directions and then use as the base for a torte. Smother in whipped cream, layer with fresh fruit, use in place of a scratch cake recipe, and go ahead and make the frosting from scratch. Box cakes, though usually unable to match the low cost of a scratch cake, can be purchased at great discounts. A box of brownie mix can also be prepared to taste like a real homemade dessert, especially when doctored with chocolate chips, syrup, and nuts.

Fruit and cake combinations are always a hit and can be thrown together at the last minute, or carefully planned and prepared. For instance, if you bake a cake that accidentally comes out of the pan in chunks, don't sweat it: break into chunks and mix with a cup or two of whipped cream. Put it into a bowl and add fresh fruit or berries, and you have a trifle.

For an easy last-minute dessert, purée 1½ cups of fruit, such as strawberries, raspberries, chopped peaches, or nectarines, with 1 cup ricotta cheese. Cut a pound of sponge cake horizontally into three layers and spread the fruit mixture between the layers and the top. Drizzle with a favorite flavored syrup and garnish with whipped cream and whole berries. Frozen raspberries or strawberries are good to use year round, when other fresh fruits are not available or economical.

As you know, ice cream is no longer made for the under-ten-year-old set. With the onslaught of gourmet ice creams in every grocery store, ice cream is a natural to end a classic gourmet meal. How about an ice cream dessert buffet for your guests? Or try serving warmed maple syrup and toasted pecans and see the reaction you'll get. Make your own premium ice cream by adding to a softened pint ½ to ¾ cup of fresh or rehydrated dried fruit, chopped nuts, any flavor crushed cookies, chocolate chips, or anything your heart desires, as the list is endless. Return to the freezer for at least 2 hours to refirm.

Ice cream pies are also fast and delicious. Bake and cool a homemade or commercial pie crust and fill with slightly softened ice cream or sherbet, mounding high in the center. Drizzle or sprinkle your favorite toppings or sauces and freeze until solid. Let stand at room temperature for 5 to 10 minutes.

After you have prepared the dessert of your choice, don't forget the garnish. Just as parsley or other garnishment adds just a little something needed on the dinner plate, dessert also needs garnishment. Fast and easy garnishes include a dollop of whipped cream and a sprig of mint, lemon or orange zest, or chocolate flakes (either white or brown).

A very impressive dessert garnish is flowers, but with a sweet twist. First make sure you're working with edible flowers (bachelor's buttons, carnations, daisies, dianthus, forget-me-nots, gardenias, honeysuckle, lilacs, marigolds, nasturtiums, pansies, impatiens, rose petals, scented geraniums, and violets). Using only flowers that you've grown yourself enables you to know they are pesticide free. Always remove the stamens and styles from the flower centers since many people are allergic to these.

Select two fresh eggs without cracks and wash gently with an anti-bacterial soap and water. Rinse well and pat dry. Separate eggs. Gently dab both sides of flowers with egg white. Sprinkle superfine granulated sugar over both sides of flowers until evenly coated. Place on wire rack and allow to dry for at least 8 hours. Use them to decorate to your heart's content.

Here's how to make gourmet coffee creamers for a fraction of the cost and calories of commercial products:

Pour one 14-ounce can fat-free sweetened condensed milk and 1½ cups skim milk into a sealable container (like a quart mason jar) that pours easily. Add the flavorings of your choice, seal, and shake vigorously or blend with a handheld immersion blender. If you add dry ingredients, such as cocoa or cinnamon, refrigerate overnight and shake again the next day to blend thoroughly.

Gourmet Coffee Creamers

Chocolate almond: 1 tablespoon cocoa powder, 1 teaspoon almond extract.

Vanilla: 2 teaspoons vanilla extract.

Strudel: 1 tablespoon cinnamon, 1 teaspoon vanilla extract, 1 teaspoon almond extract.

Cappuccino: 1 teaspoon almond extract, ½ teaspoon orange extract.

Chocolate raspberry: 2 teaspoons cocoa powder, ⅛ cup raspberry pancake syrup.

These creamers will keep until the milk's expiration date or for at least two weeks.

How to Make Espresso Drinks

Espresso: 1½ tablespoons of finely ground espresso yields one ounce of liquid, including cream. Must be brewed in an espresso maker of the pump, steam, or compression type.

Caffé Latte: Espresso with steamed milk added to fill the cup, topped with no more than ¼ inch of foam. The intensity of coffee flavor can be controlled by changing the proportions of espresso and steamed milk to taste.

Caffé Mocha: For each 8-ounce drink, coat the bottom of the cup with approximately ½ fluid ounce of chocolate syrup. Add espresso and steamed milk to fill the cup, and top with whipped cream and a sprinkle of chocolate.

Cappuccino: Espresso topped with equal parts steamed milk and foamed milk.

How to steam milk: Always use cold milk and a clean steel pitcher. Fill the pitcher ⅓ full for foaming (the milk will nearly triple in volume) and up to ⅔ full for steaming. Hold the pitcher under the steam jet of an espresso machine just beneath the surface of the milk. Heat to approximately 150° to 170° degrees to avoid scalding.

Lemon-raspberry Iced Tea

Ingredients: 16 cups water, 10 tea bags, 1½ cups sugar, 1 12-ounce bag frozen unsweetened raspberries, ¼ cup fresh lemon juice. Bring water to a boil in a large stockpot. Remove pot from heat and add all the tea bags. Let steep 3 minutes, then remove bags. Add remaining ingredients and let stand 2 to 3 minutes, stirring occasionally until raspberries have thawed. Pour tea through a fine strainer into a large pot or bowl (not aluminum) or a few large pitchers. Discard berries. Store at room temperature up to one day or refrigerate up to four days. Serve over ice.

Tips

♦ Glass bakeware conducts and retains heat better than metal, so oven temperatures should be reduced by 25 degrees whenever glass containers are used.

♦ Whipped butter contains more than 30 percent air, so it should never be used in baked goods.

♦ When baking more than one item at a time, make sure there's plenty of room between the pans, walls, and racks for air to circulate.

♦ To check whether your cake is cooking unevenly, look in 15 to 20 minutes into the baking time. If the edges look done while the center is soggy, lower the temperature by 50 degrees. You may need to increase the cooking time. Check again in 15 to 20 minutes. To correct a lopsided cake, turn the cake halfway around halfway through the cooking. Check again after 20 minutes and keep turning if necessary.

♦ Rotate baking sheets from front to back and top to bottom halfway through the baking time for more even baking.

♦ Pie crust ingredients (even flour) should be cold to produce the very best results.

♦ Sugar in a pastry dough not only contributes to its sweetness but tenderizes it as well.

♦ Body heat will melt the fat and toughen the crust, so touch the dough with your hands as little as possible.

♦ Substitute icy-cold sour cream or whipping cream for water for an extra flaky crust.

♦ Always taste the fruit before making a fruit-pie filling. If the fruit isn't sweet enough, slice it very thinly so there'll be more surfaces to absorb the sugar.

♦ When dotting the surface of a pie filling with butter, rub a cold stick of butter over the coarse side of a grater and sprinkle the grated butter over the top.

♦ Grease and flour a pie pan to prevent the crust and filling from sticking to the pan.

♦ Refrigerate leftover meringue or custard pies by covering them with plastic wrap that has been rubbed or sprayed with vegetable oil so it won't stick to the surface.

- When baking cookies, if the sheet is half or less full of cookies, it may absorb too much heat and get too hot. Place an inverted baking pan on the empty half.
- Chill the rolling pin in the freezer and the dough won't stick to it. This prevents more flour from being added to the dough.
- Most unbaked cookie dough can be refrigerated for at least a week and frozen for up to a year if wrapped airtight in freezer-weight plastic bags or foil.
- To soften a quart of rock-hard ice cream, microwave it at 30 percent power for about 30 seconds. Hardened high-fat ice cream will soften more quickly, as the microwaves are attracted to the fat.
- For ice cream that is too hard to scoop, and there's no microwave, peel away the carton and cut the ice cream into slices.
- Use nonstick vegetable spray to thinly coat ice cream scoops and spoons.
- Spray whatever container you use to melt chocolate with nonstick vegetable spray, and the melted chocolate will slip right out.
- Room temperature chocolate is easier to grate than chocolate that's too warm or too cold.
- Always defrost frozen desserts while they are still wrapped in plastic wrap. The moisture will condense on the outside of the package, not on the food.
- For a quick, cheap, and low-fat chocolate mousse: mix cocoa powder into Cool Whip. Add as little or as much cocoa powder as your palate dictates. Stir well and serve. Also can be used to frost cakes.
- Unflavored dental floss can do the job of a sharp serrated knife, and with better results. Stretched taut between your hands, a length of floss (fishing line would work too) can split a cake into layers without a turntable and with a minimum of crumbs. It also works great at slicing a log of soft fresh cheese into rounds.
- Company's coming and you're nearly out of coffee. Make mocha and you can serve 6 people with 2 cups of coffee. Add ⅓ cup

cocoa and 3 cups warmed milk to 2 cups of coffee. Sweeten to taste (about ¼ cup sugar). Add a dash of cinnamon, and you've averted a disaster!

Apple Dumplings
6 Servings

Dumplings:
- 2 cups all-purpose flour
- ¼ teaspoon salt
- ½ cup butter, cut into small pieces
- ⅔ cup sour cream
- 6 medium tart apples like pippin, cored and peeled
- ⅓ cup sugar
- ⅓ cup pecans, chopped
- 2 tablespoons butter, softened
   milk

Sauce:
- ½ cup brown sugar, firmly packed
- 2 tablespoons butter
- ½ cup whipping cream

Preheat oven to 400°. In medium-size bowl stir together flour and salt. Cut in ½ cup butter until mixture forms coarse crumbs. With fork, stir in sour cream until mixture leaves sides of bowl and forms a ball. On lightly floured surface, roll dough into 19 x 12-inch rectangle. Cut 1-inch strip of 19-inch end; reserve. Cut remaining dough into six 6-inch squares. Place an apple in the center of each square (upside down because you're going to turn it over later). In small bowl stir together sugar, pecans, and 2 tablespoons butter. Stuff about 4 teaspoons of mixture into cored center of each apple. Fold dough up around apple; seal seams well. If dough will not stick, use a little cold water as "glue." Place apples seam-side down on greased 15 x 10 x 1-inch jelly-roll pan.

Brush dough with milk and pierce dough with fork. Cut leaf designs out of reserved 1-inch strip of dough. Brush with milk; place on wrapped apples at top. Bake apples for 35 to 50 minutes until apples are fork tender. If crusts brown too quickly, cover with aluminum foil.

In a 1-quart saucepan combine all sauce ingredients. Cook over medium heat, stirring occasionally, until mixture comes to a full boil (3 to 4 minutes). Serve sauce over warm dumplings.

Nutrient value per serving: 408 calories, 6 g protein, 18 g fat, 55 g carbohydrates, 190 mg sodium, 31 mg cholesterol.

Apple Pie
6 Servings

Pastry:

1½ cups flour
1 teaspoon salt
½ cup solid vegetable shortening (Crisco)

Filling:

6 pippin apples, peeled and sliced
¾ cup sugar
2 tablespoons butter

Sift flour and salt together. Mash shortening against sides of bowl. Add 4 tablespoons ice water to make ingredients stick together. Form into ball and cut in half, roll out each, and line pie plate with one. Place sliced apples in pastry-lined pie plate. Pour sugar over apples and dot with butter. Cover with other circle of pastry, cut slits, seal, and flute. Sprinkle lightly with sugar and cinnamon. Bake 10 minutes at 450°. Decrease temperature to 350° and bake 35 to 45 minutes or until golden brown.

Nutrient value per serving: 529 calories, 4 g protein, 22 g fat, 79 g carbohydrates, 428 mg sodium, 10 mg cholesterol.

Basic Biscotti
Contributed by Betty Coates
36 Servings

I love biscotti. Whenever I have a chance to have a really good cup of coffee, I love a biscotti for dunking. However, biscotti in coffeehouses or stores is much too expensive. I have discovered that making it is not only very easy but relatively inexpensive.

1¾	cups all-purpose flour
½	teaspoon baking powder
¼	teaspoon salt
¾	cup sugar
4	tablespoons butter, chilled and cut into small pieces
1½	cups nuts (see notes)
2	large eggs
1	teaspoon flavoring (see notes)

Preheat oven to 350°. Combine flour, baking powder, salt, and sugar in food processor with metal blade. Add butter. Pulse on and off until mixture resembles cornmeal. Add nuts. Pulse about 10 times to coarsely chop.

Lightly beat together the eggs and flavoring in a small bowl. Pour evenly over the dough in the food processor and pulse the machine on and off about 20 times to moisten the dough.

Scrape the mixture onto a very lightly floured work surface. Using the heel of your hand, mash the dough with a few quick strokes to moisten any dry spots in the dough. Gather up the dough, form into a ball, then flatten into a disk. Divide the disk into 4 quarters. Form each quarter into an 8-inch long log.

Place the logs on a baking sheet that has been greased and floured about 2 inches apart. Using the heal of your hand, flatten each log so it is about 2 inches wide. Sprinkle the tops with sugar.

Bake until golden brown, about 20 minutes. Remove from the oven (leave the oven on), and using a sharp knife, cut each log on the diagonal, into about ¾-inch thick slices. Turn the biscotti cut side down on the baking sheet. Bake until they begin to color, 5 to 7 minutes. Cool on a wire rack. Store airtight.

Notes: Nuts can be any combination of your choice. The most frequently used combination is blanched almonds and toasted hazelnuts.

Flavoring can be vanilla, almond extract, or orange extract. My favorite is 2 teaspoons of anise seed.

Nutrient value per serving: 54 calories, 1 g protein, 2 g fat, 9 g carbohydrates, 38 mg sodium, 15 mg cholesterol.

Basic Sponge Cake Roll
12 Servings

When sponge cakes are used for jelly rolls, the batter is baked in a thin, even layer. Pans used for baking these cakes come in a variety of sizes, but all have sides about 1 inch high.

4	eggs, separated
⅔	cup sugar
1½	teaspoons vanilla extract
⅔	cup cake flour, sifted
1	dash salt
¼	teaspoon cream of tartar

Beat egg yolks lightly in large bowl. Add ⅓ cup sugar and continue to beat until mixture is thick and falls slowly from the beaters, leaving a ribbonlike trail. Beat in vanilla, then gently fold in flour, ⅓ cup at a time.

Using clean beaters, beat egg whites until foamy in another large bowl. Add dash of salt and cream of tartar and continue to beat until soft peaks form. Add remaining ⅓ cup sugar and beat until stiff, glossy peaks form. Gently fold egg whites into egg mixture just until no streaks remain.

Spread batter evenly in 15 x 11-inch jelly-roll pan that has been greased, floured, and lined with parchment or wax paper. Bake until top springs back when gently pressed with finger, about 15 minutes. Cool in pan for 5 minutes.

Turn cake out onto a clean kitchen towel that has been sprinkled with powdered sugar. Remove paper from bottom of cake. Trim crust on all sides with a very sharp serrated knife. Carefully roll up cake in towel so that towel is substituted for filling. Cool completely on wire rack.

When ready to fill, unroll, spread filling (such as strawberries folded into sweetened whipped cream), and carefully reroll.

Nutrient value per serving: 90 calories, 3 g protein, 12g fat, 16 g carbohydrates, 50 mg sodium, 71 mg cholesterol.

Black and White Brownies
20 Servings

Here's the most delicious, rich, moist brownie recipe you could ever hope to find. Note: Make sure you use instant coffee or instant espresso and not freeze-dried varieties.

  1   cup plus 6 tablespoons cake flour, sifted after measuring
  ½   teaspoon salt
  1   tablespoon instant coffee
  4   ounces unsweetened chocolate (baker's chocolate),
       melted and cooled to room temperature
5½   ounces unsalted butter
1½   cups white chocolate, cut up
  4   eggs
1½   cups plus 10 tablespoons sugar
  1   teaspoon vanilla extract

Preheat oven to 350°. Lightly butter and flour a 9 x 13-inch baking pan and set aside. Blend the presifted flour with salt and coffee and set aside.

In a double boiler, over medium heat, melt the baker's chocolate. When melted, add the butter and melt over low heat and stir until smooth; let cool to room temperature. (Failure to allow the chocolate to return to room temperature will result in a total flop.) While this is cooling, cut the white chocolate into bit-sized pieces. (White chocolate chips may be used if solid chocolate is not available.)

With an electric mixer, beat the eggs and sugar for about 5 minutes or until light, thick, and at the ribbon stage. Fold the room temperature–melted chocolate mixture into the eggs along with the vanilla. Gently, with a rubber spatula, fold the flour into the batter in a few smooth swift strokes. Do not overmix or the brownies will be heavy. Fold in the white chocolate chunks and transfer the batter into the prepared baking pan. Bake for about 20 to 25 minutes or until the top springs back when you press it lightly with the fingertips or when a toothpick inserted in the center of the dough comes out clean. Remove from the oven and let set until completely cool.

Cut into 20 rectangles and wrap individually in plastic wrap to keep them very fresh. May be frozen.

Nutrient value per serving: 262 calories, 38 g protein, 14 g fat, 27 g carbohydrates, 84 mg sodium, 60 mg cholesterol.

Blondies
20 Servings

3   cups flour plus 3 tablespoons flour, sifted after measuring
½   teaspoon salt
1   teaspoon baking soda
½   teaspoon baking powder
8   ounces unsalted butter
2   cups plus 10 tablespoons packed dark brown sugar
3   eggs, lightly beaten
1½ teaspoons vanilla extract
3   cups peanut butter chips (may substitute white chocolate
      OR butterscotch chips)
1   cup pecans, chopped and toasted

Preheat the oven to 350°. Lightly grease the flour in a 9 x 13-inch baking pan and set aside. Sift flour with salt, baking soda, baking powder and set aside.

Melt butter in a large saucepan over low heat. Add the brown sugar, remove it from the heat, and stir until completely blended; let cool to room temperature. Add eggs one at a time, stirring well after each addition. Stir in the vanilla.

Transfer the mixture to a large mixing bowl. With a rubber spatula, fold the sifted flour into the batter with a few smooth, swift strokes and stir just until batter is blended and smooth. Do not overmix or the blondies will be heavy.

Place pecans on a baking sheet in a 350° oven for about 10 minutes or until lightly toasted. Stir in the chips and nuts and pour batter into the prepared pan. With a spatula spread the batter to make sure it is even in thickness. Bake for 35 to 40 minutes until the top springs back when you press it lightly with your fingertips or when a toothpick inserted in the center of the dough comes out clean.

Remove the blondies from the oven and let them set until completely cool. Cut into rectangles and wrap individually in plastic wrap to keep them very fresh.

Nutrient value per serving: 247 calories, 3 g protein, 14 g fat, 27 g carbohydrates, 123 mg sodium, 57 mg cholesterol.

Carrot Cake
12 Servings

Cake:

2 cups flour, sifted
2 teaspoons baking powder
1½ teaspoons baking soda
1 teaspoon salt
2 teaspoons cinnamon
½ cup walnuts, chopped
1 cup golden raisins, optional
2 cups sugar
4 eggs
1½ cups oil
2 cups carrots, grated raw
1 8½ ounce size can crushed pineapple, drained

Frosting:

½ cup butter, softened
1 8 ounce size cream cheese, softened
1 teaspoon vanilla
1 1 pound box powdered sugar, sifted

Sift flour again with baking powder, baking soda, salt, and cinnamon. Set aside. Beat eggs lightly in separate bowl and stir into oil. Add with sugar to flour mixture. Stir in carrots, drained pineapple, nuts, and raisins.

Pour into 3 greased and floured 8-inch cake pans. Bake at 350° oven for 35 to 40 minutes. Cool 10 minutes and remove from pan. Cool completely before frosting.

Frosting: Combine butter, cream cheese, and vanilla, and cream well. Add sugar gradually, beating well.

Nutrient value per serving: 638 calories, 6 g protein, 7 g fat, 64 g carbohydrates, 464 mg sodium, 92 mg cholesterol.

Chocolate Mint Mousse
4 Servings

6	ounces semisweet chocolate
3	eggs, separated
1 to 2	tablespoons sugar
¾	cup heavy cream
½	teaspoon mint extract
	whipped cream, for garnish
	fresh mint, for garnish

Melt the chocolate in a double boiler over simmering water. Remove from the heat and pour into a mixing bowl. Lightly beat the egg yolks and blend them into the chocolate.

In a separate bowl beat the egg whites to a soft peak. Add sugar and beat again to form stiff peaks.

Mix a third of the whites into the chocolate mixture and then fold the chocolate into the remaining beaten whites, a little at a time.

Whip the heavy cream with the mint extract until stiff, and fold into the chocolate mixture. Chill thoroughly. Garnish with whipped cream and fresh mint leaves.

Nutrient value per serving: 505 calories, 8 g protein, 39 g fat, 31 g carbohydrates, 84 mg sodium, 232 mg cholesterol.

Classic Cheesecake
16 Servings

Crust:
1½ cups graham cracker crumbs
6 tablespoons butter, melted
½ cup walnuts, chopped

Filling:
2 8 ounce packages cream cheese, softened at room
   temperature
1 cup sugar
2 eggs
1 pint sour cream
1 teaspoon vanilla extract

Preheat oven to 350°.

To prepare crust, stir together graham cracker crumbs, butter, and nuts. Press over bottom and sides of an 8 x 8 x 2-inch cake pan.

Filling: In a large bowl thoroughly beat together cream cheese and sugar; beat in eggs one at a time, then sour cream and vanilla until well blended.

Pour into prepared crust and bake in 350° oven for 35 minutes. Turn oven off, open the door, and allow cake to stand in the oven for 1 hour longer. Chill.

Note: Because of the nature of cream cheese, this cheesecake must be made 24 hours in advance of serving.

Nutrient value per serving: 322 calories, 51 g protein, 24 g fat, 21 g carbohydrates, 202 mg sodium, 81 mg cholesterol.

Flowerpots
24 Servings

24 small flower pots, thoroughly cleaned
½ gallon chocolate burnt-almond ice cream
½ gallon coffee ice cream
1½ cups favorite flavored syrup
1 package chocolate wafer cookies, crumbled finely

Fill pots halfway with chocolate burnt-almond ice cream. Fill almost to top with coffee ice cream, then pour 1 tablespoon of your favorite flavored syrup on top. Sprinkle with crumbled wafers to fill. Freeze.

Remove from freezer prior to serving to thaw slightly. Stick flower and fern in for visual effect (or gummy worms, if they're for kids).

Glazed Fresh Strawberry Pie
6 Servings

1 pastry crust, baked and cooled
6 cups fresh strawberries, washed and hulled
1 cup sugar
3½ tablespoons cornstarch
½ cup water
red food coloring

½ pint whipping cream
1 tablespoon sugar
½ teaspoon vanilla extract

Separate berries, leaving 4 cups whole, and mash or purée the remaining 2 cups. Mix sugar and cornstarch in a 3-quart saucepan. Stir in water and puréed berries. Cook over medium heat, stirring constantly until mixture comes to a full boil. Boil 2 minutes, stirring constantly. If color is not vibrant red, add red food coloring until desired color is achieved. Remove from heat. Place a piece of cheesecloth inside a large sieve and strain the liquid into a large bowl. Allow to come to room temperature. Once cooled, gently fold remaining whole berries into the glaze. Pile into pastry shell. Chill well.

Whip cream until soft peaks form. Gradually add sugar and vanilla and continue beating until desired consistency is achieved.

Serve pie with whipped cream.

Nutrient Value Per Serving: 624 calories, 4 g protein, 25 g fat, 95 g carbohydrates, 201 mg sodium, 54 mg cholesterol.

Lemon Cake
16 Servings

 1 package yellow cake mix
 4 eggs
 ¾ cup vegetable oil
 ¾ cup water
 1 teaspoon lemon extract
 1 3 ounce package lemon gelatin

Glaze:
 1 cup powdered sugar
 3 tablespoons lemon juice

Preheat oven to 350°. Lightly butter and flour a 9 x 13-inch baking pan. Mix all cake ingredients well following the mixing time recommended on box. Pour into the prepared baking pan and bake for about 35 to 40 minutes. Test for doneness by inserting a toothpick into the center of the cake. If it comes out clean, the cake is done.

Glazing: Mix powdered sugar and lemon juice. Spread over hot cake.

When cake is cool, cut into pieces and serve.

Nutrient value per serving: 143 calories, 2 g protein, 11 g fat, 8 g carbohydrates, 17 mg sodium, 53 mg cholesterol.

Lemon Meringue Pie
Contributed by Jan Sandberg
6 Servings

Crust:
2   cups flour
1   cup solid vegetable shortening (Crisco is best)
1   teaspoon salt
5 to 6   tablespoons ice water

Filling:
2   cups water
4 to 5   tablespoons cornstarch
1½   cups sugar
¼   teaspoon salt
4   egg yolks
¼   cup fresh lemon juice
3   tablespoons butter

Meringue:
8   tablespoons sugar
4   egg whites
¼   teaspoon cream of tartar

Crust: Preheat oven to 400°. Sift flour and salt together. Mash Crisco with fork or pastry cutter into flour mixture. Mix ice water with mixture until it sticks together. Roll out and put in pie plate. Prick with fork on bottom and sides. Bake 12 to 15 minutes. While baking, make filling.

Filling: In a medium saucepan dissolve cornstarch in water; add egg yolks, sugar, salt, and lemon juice. Beat with rotary beater to blend. Cook to just boiling point and add butter. Pour into baked pie shell. While cooling, make meringue.

Meringue: In a clean bowl with clean beaters, beat egg whites and cream of tartar at high speed until soft peaks form. Gradually add sugar, one tablespoon at a time. Beat until soft and glossy. Spread over pie filling, making sure it touches pastry shell all the way around and no lemon filling is exposed. Pile high in the center. Bake in 350° oven for 12 to 15 minutes or until meringue just starts to brown.

Nutrient value per serving: 977 calories, 9 g protein, 44 g fat, 137 g carbohydrates, 887 mg sodium, 152 mg cholesterol.

Pumpkin Pie
6 Servings

¾ cup sugar
1 teaspoon cinnamon
1 teaspoon ginger
½ teaspoon salt
1½ cups pumpkin purée, made from fresh pumpkin,
   instructions to follow
3 eggs
¾ cup evaporated milk
¾ cup water
1 unbaked pie shell

To prepare puréed pumpkin: Cut pumpkin open and remove all membranes, strings, and seeds. Cut into small wedges and steam in large vegetable steamer until fork-tender. Remove from steamer and cool overnight in the refrigerator. Scoop out meat from rind and place in blender or food processor. Process on purée setting until smooth. Line a colander with cheesecloth, place puréed pumpkin in colander, and allow to drain until all visible liquid has stopped dripping out.

Place sugar, spices, and salt in large bowl and blend well. Add puréed pumpkin and blend well with electric mixer on medium speed. Add beaten eggs, milk, and water. Continue mixing until well blended. Pour into prepared pie shell. Bake at 425° until crust begins to brown (about 15 minutes). Lower heat to 350° and continue baking until set (about 30 minutes). Test doneness by inserting toothpick in center. If pick comes out clean, pumpkin is set.

Nutrient value per serving: 221 calories, 6 g protein, 5 g fat, 37 g carbohydrates, 263 mg sodium, 116 mg cholesterol.

Six-Layer Toffee Torte
20 Servings

2⅔ cups all-purpose flour
2 cups sugar
1 cup butter (2 sticks), softened
1 cup buttermilk
¾ cup cocoa
2 teaspoons baking soda
1½ teaspoons vanilla extract
¼ teaspoon salt
2 eggs
2½ teaspoons instant coffee granules
10 chocolate toffee bars, 1.4 ounces each
2 cups heavy cream
3 tablespoons light brown sugar

About 3 hours before serving or early in the day: Preheat oven to 350°. Grease and flour three 8-inch round cake pans.

Into a large bowl measure the first nine ingredients. With electric mixer at low speed, beat ingredients until just mixed, constantly scraping bowl with rubber spatula. Dissolve 2 teaspoons instant coffee in 1 cup boiling water; add to bowl. Increase speed to medium; beat 2 minutes, occasionally scraping bowl.

Pour batter into pans. Bake 25 to 30 minutes until toothpick inserted in center of cake comes out clean. Cool cake in pans on wire racks 10 minutes. Remove from pans; cool completely on racks.

While cake is cooling, finely chop toffee bars. In cup dissolve ½ teaspoon instant coffee in 1 teaspoon hot water. Cool.

With serrated knife, cut each cake layer horizontally in half to make 6 thin layers. In large bowl, with mixer at medium speed, beat heavy (whipping) cream, brown sugar, and dissolved instant coffee until stiff peaks form.

To assemble cake, place 1 layer on cake plate; spread with about ½ cup whipped-cream mixture. Reserve about two-thirds of finely chopped toffee bars; sprinkle layer with about one-fifth of remaining finely chopped toffee bars. Repeat layering 4 more times; top with remaining cake layer. Thinly spread remaining whipped-cream mixture over side and top of cake. Gently press reserved toffee bars onto side and top of cake. Refrigerate cake until ready to serve. Serves 20.

Nutrient value per serving: 447 calories, 5 g protein, 26 g fat, 48 g carbohydrates, 271 mg sodium, 54 mg cholesterol.

Part Three

Presenting the Pleasures of the Table

Style has nothing to do with money.
Anybody can do it with money.
The true art is to do it on a shoestring.
—Tom Hogan

Chapter 15

*J*ust Another
Ordinary Meal or a
Memorable Occasion?

A gourmet meal combines the pleasure of eating with the
physical participation of others. A gourmet meal can be one
where the talents, enthusiasm, and creativity of the cook are
even more important to the guests than the actual food that is
served. This meal is not pretentious and results
in a lovely shared experience.
—Nancy Guth

Now that you've mastered the planning and creation of a meal, there is one more very important element, the presentation of your work. Yes, that's right; next to the actual taste and quality of the food, nothing will affect the outcome of a meal more than where and how it is served. And believe me, that can swing either way too. Serve up a plain casserole on nice dishes with a linen tablecloth and I bet anything that your family will react differently than if you served it family style with paper napkins and the television on. Add a sprig of parsley, require them to wash their hands and put on a clean shirt, and you can transform mealtime at your home. And what did it cost you? A little extra for the bunch of parsley and a little elbow grease getting the dust off those nice dishes.

I know it's worth it in my home. The reaction I get from Harold and my two boys when I present dinner with a little extra flair is well worth the tiny bit of effort on my part. And do you know why? It's because it tells them that I value them, that I value our time together, that they're special. When a family member or friend who is dining at your home feels a sense of belonging and value, you have accomplished more than just creating a good meal. That is what entertaining and the comfort of good food provides.

A gourmet meal doesn't have to mean small portions with decorative sauce squirted all around the plate. Presentation is very important. A pot roast with colorful veggies and beautifully whipped potatoes is considered a gourmet meal in my home.

—Mary Ann Woirhaye

When planning a dinner party or get-together, most of us spend all of our energies, budget, and time on the actual menu, which for obvious reasons is well placed. However, presentation doesn't cost anything but adds everything. You are creating an atmosphere, an ambiance to match your menu and the personalities of your guests. This is where imagination and creativity come in handy. And for those of you that are creatively challenged, get yourself to a library or newsstand and start looking through magazines, or turn on the food channel and start taking notes on presentation. There is a reason that magazines pay big bucks for creative consultants, decorators, and food stylists. If you like what you see, then chances are you'll keep referring to their publication for information and ideas. You benefit because you're getting ideas from experts that have spent a lot of time experimenting to create a "look."

The sky is the limit when it comes to presentation. You've already accomplished the major portion of the event—the food. Now it's time to finish the job.

The Atmosphere

Where you choose to serve your meal has a lot to do with the happiness of your guests. The size of the room, its ventilation, and proximity to the kitchen should all be considered when deciding how many guests to invite and where you will actually feed them. A wonderful gourmet meal doesn't disappoint the tastebuds, but it also creates a mood, and the atmosphere must match that mood. Short of buying a new house or having your furniture recovered, think outside the lines and perhaps move your meal to another room. Perhaps an intimate dinner in front of the fireplace with the lights low, the glow of the fire and candles providing both warmth and light.

If you have one of those wonderfully large kitchens, create a farmhouse effect with everyone dining in the kitchen, with the aroma of the food delighting the senses and everyone sharing in the event. A kitchen creates a sense of security; it is the heart and soul of many households, and it's no surprise we love to congregate in the kitchen. It can be creatively decorated with lots of candles, arrangements of wild flowers and greens, and the displaying of some of your more unusual serving pieces. The great thing about entertaining in the kitchen is that your menu and the mood can be more casual. (You might want to clean off the front of the fridge first!)

The Room

When guests arrive, whether you birthed them or they are official "dinner guests," they always walk into your home and look around the room. And if they are of the male persuasion, they are on the lookout for food. Now, keeping in mind that having food tells them you think they are special, you better have some ready. First impressions say a lot, and don't be discouraged if the first thing they see isn't the beautiful flower arrangement you put together yourself or the creatively set table. Whatever puts them at ease and makes them feel welcome is what you're after, right? A hands-down favorite at my house for creating that wonderful feeling is the aroma of baking bread. If you're not a bread baker, some wonderful frozen breads are available in the market, and they smell and taste great.

Be creative in how you serve your appetizers. Since you are not having to limit your serving pieces to the confines of your table, serve chips and popcorn in big baskets, or how about in the brim of a sombrero or cowboy hat. A little different perhaps, but you will have left a creative memory for your guests. And don't forget to add some visuals to your appetizer table. Whether it's a simple arrangement of greenery, a grouping of some collectibles you have, or a splash of color using linens, each food area needs your attention because that's where your guests will congregate.

The Table

For a sit-down meal, the table is the focus for the evening. I have gone to dinner parties where twelve people sat glued to their chairs talking, laughing, and eating for three to four hours without moving other than to help the hostess clear the dishes. If your goal is to make entertaining a priority, a large table with comfortable chairs should be on your list to acquire someday.

It is because of this fascination of ours to sit at the table for hours that the presentation of the table should be appealing, inviting, and comfortable. First, let's talk about how many can sit comfortably around your table. Think about that and then admit that unless you've invited sardines to your dinner party no one wants to be greased up and stuffed into their seat. Until Harold and I created Big Table, we were limited to ten. That was it, and I knew it. Realize what your limit is and stick with it.

Now, depending on the theme of your party—casual or formal, holiday or any day—you will create the visuals on your table around that theme. This is where so many hostesses get in trouble because they think they have to spend lots of money on flowers, linens, and other accessories. Wrong. Our panelist Paulette Hegg sums up table presentation the best: "I don't have an open-ended food budget, so I feel it's a gift from myself to my family and guests to make the food and table look good even if the meal by some standards is not gourmet."

Homegrown flowers and herbs add a lot of color, and adding different shapes and sizes of candles creates a very inviting table. I am convinced that ivy was God's decorating gift to the dinner party hostess. I am among the millions of Americans who have ivy growing in my yard, and I use it abundantly in my decorating. Whether it lines a tray of appetizers, snakes through the candles on the table, or serves as a place card (yes, that's right—write your guests' names on a big green leaf of ivy with those metallic pens), it adds more than a standard bouquet of flowers ever could. And the best part is—it's free! If you don't have ivy, I encourage you to make friends with your neighbor who does.

The Plate

Finally, we come to what you've worked so hard for, the fruits of your labor. There is an old adage about food that is so true: "You eat with your eyes first." A simple but deft finishing touch can turn a visually neutral dish into one that's smashing. Garnishes add eye appeal and don't have to be time-consuming or put a strain on your budget. There is a rule of thumb, however, and that is that any garnish should be edible and when possible, an ingredient that complements the dish. Keeping that in mind will make it easy to add garnishes. Just buy a little or snip a little extra of that herb, vegetable, or fruit for your garnish.

Another way to make your plate visually appealing is by being a little creative or different in the way a dish is displayed on the plate. Put mashed potatoes in your pastry bag and squeeze for presentation. Experiment with other utensils you might have. Use a citrus stripper to flute mushrooms by carving out strips at even intervals. Present soups or stews in bowls lined with lettuce or spinach. Make scalloped edges in citrus fruits, experiment with flower radishes, and so on.

The only limit on how your food is prepared is your imagination. Try serving your meal in courses instead of all at once. This lengthens your evening and really places the emphasis during the meal on the food. Whatever you choose to do, however, the most important thing is for you to be relaxed and enthusiastic and for your guests to crave a return invitation.

> *Gourmet food is pleasing in taste, texture, and presentation. When someone first sees it, they should say, "This looks delicious!" When they first taste it, they should stop for a moment, roll their eyes toward heaven, and say, "This is wonderful!" When they are finished, they should feel satisfied, have a smile on their face, and not be so full that they are miserable.*
> —Deborah Taylor Hough

$\mathcal{T}$he Ultimate in Cheapskate Hospitality and Entertaining

*Come and share a pot of tea, my home is warm and my
friendship's free.*
—Emilie Barnes

Once you have achieved confidence in the preparation and presentation of fine food, a desire to entertain and share your accomplishments with friends and family will be a natural outgrowth. The problem for many is not having the desire to entertain but in finding a way to handle the expense of such an endeavor.

Most of us live according to a spending plan or some kind of budget which requires that either the additional cost of the event be covered by the weekly or monthly food allowance or that the necessary funds be diverted from some other expense category. In the case of working the additional expense into the regular food allowance, one may need to spread the cost of the dinner party over several weeks or months. Of course it would be advisable to plan far enough ahead to allow ample time to save the required funds.

There's no denying that entertaining has a cost. However, there are many creative ways one can keep that cost way down by simply thinking outside the lines—breaking the "rules" if necessary.

Following are suggestions for two economical ways to entertain.

The first is very elegant and exquisite; the second, more casual and fun. Let your mind wander, and you'll begin thinking of ways you can adapt these ideas to your own situation.

A British Cream Tea

Recently I hosted my second afternoon British cream tea. A friend and I cohosted the first tea, which was a baby shower for my friend and colleague, Cathy Hollenbeck. We had about twelve guests, and it turned out very successfully. It was so well received and remembered, I felt confident in repeating the idea.

This time it was a bridal tea (instead of the traditional bridal shower), honoring my friend Nancy Chapman, who was to be married four weeks hence.

I will describe the tea in every detail, assuming that you may want to adapt such an event to your own situation. Keep in mind my two major areas of concern: First, I did not want to include anything the guests might expect at a traditional wedding shower, i.e., games, cake, coordinated paper goods, honeycomb and crepe paper decorations, etc. Second, I needed to keep the costs of hosting this affair as low as possible. This was to be an economical and exquisite event—chic and cheap!

A British cream tea is as elegant and inviting as it sounds and offers a wonderful and inexpensive opportunity to entertain in the afternoon between traditional mealtimes. A tea is perfect for a no-occasion celebration, a friendly get-together, birthday party, bridal or baby shower, and can be adapted for as few as four guests or as many as thirty-five—possibly more.

I fudged a bit by calling this 2:00 P.M. affair high tea. According to the strictest of British tradition, high tea should commence after 4:30 in the afternoon. I did as I encourage you to do—customize and take reasonable risks. As it turns out, no one noticed (or had the heart to point out) my intentional faux pas.

While most teas are hosted for small groups, this particular bridal shower had a long guest list that resulted in thirty-five confirmed attendees. I wanted very much for the group to gather in one place so that all could be seated at the bride-to-be's table. I wanted my guests to be pampered to the hilt, which eliminated any thought of serving buffet style. Small tables scattered throughout the house would defeat my purpose of intimacy. Can you imagine thirty-five people trying to walk around while maneuvering plates of food and cups of hot tea?

I commenced with the planning about one month before the big day. First I collected books from the library and friends to learn all I could about British teas. This was going to be as authentic as I could manage, and to my amazement, I had a lot to learn.

I made the invitations with my computer and laser printer and printed them on paper stock I had on hand. I chose plain paper, used a very readable script font, and included no graphics or pictures. Simple elegance. This method was far less expensive and far more beautiful than purchasing manufactured invitations. A copy follows:

When Anna, the seventh Duchess of Bedford, made her first eloquent request for afternoon refreshment, she started a tradition that is still beloved a century and a half later. The British Cream Tea is the epitome of this afternoon pleasure.

A Cream Tea is so called because it is just that, a tea with clotted cream and the products of milk: butter, whipped cream, and custards. These and a wonderful array of sandwiches, scones, cookies, cakes, and pastries grace the Tea table.

Mind you, the British do not indulge in a Cream Tea every afternoon. When the British do a Cream Tea, it's heaven, as it will be for us when on

Saturday, the Twenty-third Day of March at two o'clock in the afternoon

We will shower gifts and best wishes on

Lady Nancy Kathleen, Princess of the House of Chapman

upon the occasion of her impending nuptials.

> *The pleasure of your company is requested at that time*
> *and date*
>
> *The House of Hunt, My Address, City, and State*
>
> *You are invited to attire yourself in afternoon elegance as*
> *would be fitting for*
>
> *High Tea with a Princess*

Enclosed with each invitation was a reply postcard, postage-paid, (at that time, 22-cents for a reply in an envelope), also made on my computer.

My next challenge was the tea table, place settings, and seating. I don't know too many people who just happen to have a table and sufficient elegant serving pieces to entertain groups of thirty-five.

The Table

I hoped that once I figured out this central item, everything would fall into place. Harold made me a big table several years ago for holiday dining. It is exquisite and so useful. He took two 8-feet by 4-feet sheets of ¾-inch plywood and joined them by screwing several 3-inch by ¾-inch flat joining bars (about 50 cents each at the home center) and attached them on the underside where the two pieces join. The result was one continuous tabletop 16 feet long by 4 feet wide.

I named her Big Table. She sits on two regular tables (my dining table and a metal folding table) that are positioned about four feet in from either end and act as massive "pedestals." I know you can't imagine this, but it is very sturdy, strong, and does not cause a guest to feel anxious that the whole thing just might flip up and toss everyone into the next room. When not in use, Big Table is unassembled and screwed right to the wall of our garage.

Because Big Table is so much wider than the supporting pedestals, no one has to straddle a leg, which increases the seating capacity and comfort.

Because five people can sit comfortably on either side of each eight-foot sheet of plywood and two can sit at each end, Big Table can easily accommodate twenty-four. But thirty-five would be out of the question. My solution for the tea was to get one more piece of plywood and a third table pedestal, which would expand Big Table to twenty-four feet in length; enough room for thirty-four. Since the group would include several young ladies, I was fairly confident I could find a way to squeeze in one more little person, which I did.

Because our dining room/living room area is straight (not L-shaped) and measures thirty feet in length, Big Table at her greatest expanse would slip into the space with enough room to maneuver around the end chairs. However, this new configuration would allow for precious few other pieces of furniture in the room. The dining table was in use as a pedestal so everything else was easily relocated to other rooms except for my favorite possession, my six-foot grand piano.

We moved the piano into the entry area where, thankfully, it fit perfectly and remains to this day. With the lid opened, a big bouquet of flowers, and a silver candelabra, I decided this would make a striking statement as guests arrived.

Dressing Big Table

Take a moment to envision one continuous table 24 feet long by 4 feet wide. That's 96 square feet, or 13,824 square inches! Unfortunately, unfinished plywood doesn't go well with English bone china and needs to be covered.

Several years ago I purchased four flat twin-sized sheets in dark green for Big Table. They cost six dollars each and would be used as table coverings exclusively. Laid end to end, four of them (overlapped) fit extra-large Big Table perfectly, including a six-inch drop all the way around. Dark green is a great winter color but not too exciting for a spring bridal tea. I had to find something charming yet cheap to accommodate her 30 percent growth. I was thinking of a table topper or skirt.

I considered flowered sheets (I couldn't find anything affordable) and yard goods (this would require too many seams and about 20 yards of fabric—ouch!). My friend Rosalie suggested we check out Marshall's, a large name-brand outlet. We struck pure gold in a back corner of the store under piles of mismatched linens. There they were, four Battenburg lace tablecloths, each 120 inches by 72-inches. Perfect size. The bonus was the twelve matching napkins included with each tablecloth. At fifteen dollars for each cloth and twelve napkins, it was a bargain I could not pass up.

Desperate, I rummaged through my stash of yard goods and blessed the day I picked up two king-size sheets in a beautiful flowered motif. The colors were perfect and now I was mighty thankful I'd purchased them many years before.

Before you faint from shock, remember Big Table is made of plywood, is very rugged, and is not too pretty in her undressed state. I cut the flowered sheets into 18-inch strips, hemmed one of the long sides, then pleated and stapled it (yes, you read that right) all around the 56-foot perimeter. I then placed the dark green sheets on the top (ironed them right in place on the table) and topped them with the Battenburg cloths. The dark green peeked through all the beautiful cut-work. The white coverings dropped about six inches leaving twelve inches of the flowered skirt showing. It was a perfect tea length.

Once the table was properly dressed for the occasion, everything else fell into place, and quite inexpensively. When my friends heard of my ambitious undertaking, offers of china, teapots, plates, flatware, vases, and everything one could ever imagine came flooding my way. Clearly many people like myself have lovely things that are kept in a cupboard to collect dust.

I used gorgeous pieces I'd had for twenty-five years and which had never been used. What a shame.

My biggest fear was not breaking things (although that was a concern); it was comingling everything and then not being able to remember what belongs to whom. I would be responsible to return each precious piece to its owner. My solution: As I accepted pieces, I immediately polished and washed them and then color-coded each piece by sticking a colored dot (available at stationery stores) representing that person on the bottom. Now I was free to mix and match everything without worry. Just envision thirty-five cups and saucers each in a different pattern, seventy luncheon plates, and thirty-five place-settings of silver flatware, not to mention all the teapots, crystal pitchers, water goblets, and serving pieces. I'm not sure I could have picked my own from the group.

The contributions of seven people plus myself produced enough gorgeous English bone china teapots, serving trays, cream and sugar sets, flatware, water goblets, and various small bowls (even a silver tea service and antique tea cart). Each group of four guests had (in addition to their own teacup, saucer, unique teaspoon, flatware, and water goblet) a teapot, creamer and sugar, and serving trays to share between them. This would eliminate the need to pass things, which I prayed would reduce the chance of untimely accidents.

The Centerpiece

I gathered my nonmatching crystal stemware (don't we all have these odd pieces hanging around?) of all heights and shapes in a random grouping for the center and allowed them to trail off about a foot in either direction. The centerpiece measured four-feet in length, total. Each goblet was filled partially with water and a white floating candle.

I included several other crystal pieces other than stemware in the centerpiece to achieve the look I wanted (a taller vase in the center and short crystal bowls and dishes at the ends). Now it wasn't so much the same and was a very interesting collection of shapes and heights. I intertwined the crystal bases with fresh large-leafed ivy (plucked from my yard) and allowed the ivy to wind its way right to the far ends of the center table section. I scattered tiny fuschia-colored blooms and baby's breath on the ivy and dropped a few of the smallest blooms into the goblets where they floated on the water and encircled the floating candles.

Because the odd crystal glasses and goblets, and champagnes were of varying heights and facets (about twenty pieces total), once lighted, the arrangement was glorious even in the daylight.

Each person's teacup and saucer matched with no duplicates at the table. Beyond that I mixed all the pieces, and it was breathtakingly beautiful. I folded each new Battenburg lace napkin into a rose (napkin-folding books are easily found). My friend Mary Ann Woirhaye contributed thirty-five matching bone china nameplates onto which I wrote each person's first name (it washes right off for the next use). Gorgeous patterns of silver flatware gave the finishing touch.

This entire table setting for thirty-five cost four dollars, the cost of the floating candles. (I did not include the additional table top, tablecloths, and napkins in the cost because they were not single-use, and I will gladly add them to my personal inventory to be used in the future). Had I gone the expensive way and purchased high-quality single-use paper plates, cups, napkins, tablecloths, etc., the cost would have been closer to two dollars per person.

Because of the large group and the need for some kind of conformity I rented matching white cafe chairs for the occasion. I breathed a sign of relief as thirty-five of them fit perfectly around Big Table.

I made a trip to a local wholesale flower warehouse late the day before the event and picked up large bunches of whatever had not sold earlier in the day. The prices were slashed because of the late hour. I arranged beautiful spring flowers into large bouquets and placed them throughout the house and patio. They looked as if they'd just been cut from Martha's garden rather than stiffly arranged with oasis, wire, and bows. The sweet peas, snap dragons, daffodils, hyacinths, wax flowers, and baby's breath contributed a delicate, sweet fragrance. With the windows opened and a lovely sea breeze filling the house, it was hard to believe I wasn't sitting in an authentic English garden.

The Food

All of the food was homemade in the two days prior to The Day (except for the imported tea biscuits) and served in three courses:

FIRST COURSE
Cucumber Sandwiches*
Chicken Almond Salad Sandwiches*
Curried-Egg Salad Sandwiches*
Fresh Fruits of the Season

SECOND COURSE
Scones*
Raspberry Preserves
Clotted Cream*

THIRD COURSE
Lemon Petticoat Tails*
Pecan Tartlettes*
Black Raspberry Preserves–Filled Shortbread*
White Chocolate–Dipped Strawberries
Chocolate-covered English Tea Biscuits

*Recipes follow.

The menu was printed on a small "program" which was placed on each plate and also included some tea trivia and personal messages. I included acknowledgment of those who had lent their treasures as follows: "Most of the items on today's tea table belong to the hostess. The balance are on loan from the private collections of . . ." That sounded better to me than thanking people for letting me borrow their stuff.

Three of my friends volunteered to help prepare the food and serve the tea. They wore plain black skirts and blouses and matching Battenburg aprons which added to the authenticity and uniqueness of the occasion. All of the guests were dressed beautifully; some wore hats and gloves.

The Tea

Once everyone was seated, I asked each person to give their name and briefly tell the group how they knew Nancy and when they first met. This broke the ice and relieved everyone's curiosity since a lot of the guests were from the future bridegroom's family whom many of us had not met. This allowed Nancy to relax and assisted me as the hostess to make everyone feel welcome.

During the self-introductions, Cathy, Kelly, and Rosalie brought in steaming pots of tea. As the introductions concluded, they began serving the first course, which had been beautifully arranged on individual clear glass luncheon plates. These were placed directly on each person's china plate.

Once the first course was consumed, the servers picked up the plates and returned with the second course: warmed scones served on nine trays and placed about the table. Each group of four guests had their own bowls of clotted cream, strawberry preserves, and scones. Tea cups were refilled as necessary until time for the third course, dessert.

By now the clear glass plates which were picked up from the first course had been washed and individually filled with an array of colorful and gorgeous desserts.

The food not only looked wonderful, it was absolutely delicious. And there was so much of it. Guests were relaxed and comfortable enough at the close of the dessert course to ask for a sandwich bag to take home any items they could not eat. What a great idea and high compliment, and I cheerfully handed out small zip-type bags which we called, appropriately, "tea bags."

Serving of the tea in three courses took nearly two hours. This was plenty of time to relax and leisurely enjoy the setting and the company.

The ladies were then invited to take a powder-room break and retire to the family room where the presents were waiting. Everyone found a comfortable place to sit, and Nancy began opening the many gifts.

The entire tea lasted three and a half hours, and everything went perfectly. I attribute the success to detailed and early planning and the generous assistance of my friends. While there were accolades and compliments on the events of the afternoon, I believe the most surprising came from one of the guests who slipped into the kitchen and asked my hard-working friends for a business card. She assumed they were from a catering company and couldn't bear the thought of not knowing how to reach them in the future.

Guests thanked me for not subjecting them to silly games, and I am certain no one missed the traditional sheet cake. On the contrary, many expressed their thankfulness for having been included and promised this was a bridal shower they would never forget. I'll second the motion.

Suggestions for Adapting a British Cream Tea

Borrow as many serving pieces, table coverings, teacups, and so on as possible. I was surprised how many felt honored to have their possessions used for such a classy event. Nothing was broken and everything promptly returned to its rightful owner. I had the offer of far more beautiful things than I could ever have used. Design your table to fit your room. If you think "modularly," the idea of building tabletops may provide the solution you need.

Select flowers which grow prolifically in your area. Your neighbors and friends will likely enjoy contributing cuttings from their yards. If your event is in winter, use various evergreen branches to decorate; in autumn pull in all kinds of fall leaves, pods, and dried flowers. In the summer most areas are blessed with roses, chrysanthemums, and gladioli.

Simplify or expand the menu as you like. If you are short on free time, select items which can be prepared ahead and frozen until the day.

Brew the tea in your kitchen rather than introducing tea bags or tea balls to the tea table. I served only one type of tea (Barry's Gold Blend), which eliminated taking orders and having to look at unsightly used tea bags.

Before you purchase anything, spend time thinking of ways you can avoid doing so. Other than ingredients for the menu and postage for the invitations, you should be able to get by without spending much money.

Clearly, what this kind of entertaining lacks in expense it more than makes up in time and effort required. But isn't the whole point of entertaining to give of yourself, not necessarily your means? For me this event was the very highest expression of love and best wishes I could have ever given to Nancy, the oldest child of our friends Duane and Kathleen Chapman and whom I have known since nine months before her birth.

Black Raspberry Preserves–Filled Shortbread
36 Servings

1½ cups butter, softened
2   teaspoons vanilla
3   cups all-purpose flour, sifted
1½ cups powdered sugar, sifted
    seedless black raspberry preserves

Preheat oven to 325°.

Cream butter in medium bowl with electric mixer set at medium speed. Add powdered sugar and beat until smooth. Add vanilla and mix until creamy. Scrape bowl. Add flour and mix at low speed until thoroughly mixed. Gather dough into two balls and flatten to disks. Wrap dough tightly in plastic wrap, or place in airtight plastic food bag. Refrigerate one hour or until firm.

Using floured rolling pin, roll dough onto floured board to ¼-inch thickness. Cut out 2-inch hearts with cookie cutters. Continue using dough scraps, rerolling and recutting until all dough is used. Be careful not to overwork dough.

Place cookies on ungreased baking sheet, ½ inch apart. Bake for 16 to 18 minutes or until firm. Transfer to cool, flat surface with spatula.

Spread black raspberry preserves on the bottom side of half the baked and cooled cookies. Top jam-spread cookies with bottom side of remaining cookies, forming sandwiches. If desired, sift powdered sugar over finished cookies.

Nutrient value per serving: 107 calories, 1 g protein, 8 g fat, 8 g carbohydrates, 78 mg sodium, 21 mg cholesterol.

Chicken-Almond Dill Sandwiches
24 Servings

       3 chicken breasts, cooked and finely chopped
      ¾ cup slivered almonds, finely chopped
      ½ cup mayonnaise
1 to 2 tablespoons dried dill weed (not dill seeds)
          salt and pepper to taste
          unsalted butter
     12 slices white bread

Combine all ingredients and mix well. Spread the bread slices with a thin coating of butter to seal the bread so it does not become soggy. Spread ½ of chicken mixture on each slice and spread evenly. With a sharp serrated knife, trim away all crusts. Cut slices into two or four pieces. Garnish with a small sprig of fresh dill.

Nutrient value per serving: 146 calories, 9 g protein, 8 g fat, 8 g carbohydrates, 165 mg sodium, 22 mg cholesterol.

Clotted Cream
6 Servings

The cream used in England is generally unavailable in this country. However, we clever Americans have come up with several reasonable facsimiles, and this is definitely one of the best!

     1 cup heavy cream, at room temperature
    ⅓ cup sour cream, at room temperature
     1 tablespoon powdered sugar

Must be made at least one hour before serving. Pour the heavy cream into a bowl and beat until soft peaks form. Whisk in the sour cream and sugar, continuting to beat until the mixture is very thick. Cover and place in refrigerator until time to serve. You can make this ahead, provided it is used within 6 hours.

Nutrient value per serving: 174 calories, 1 g protein, 17 g fat, 3 g carbohydrates, 20 mg sodium, 60 mg cholesterol.

Cucumber Sandwiches
12 Servings

½ cucumber, peeled and thinly sliced
1 tablespoon sugar
1 tablespoon apple cider vinegar
   unsalted butter
6 slices white bread
   salt and pepper to taste

Combine the cucumber, sugar, and vinegar in a bowl. Toss to blend. Allow to sit for ½ hour. Drain off excess liquid. Spread a thin coating of butter on each slice of bread (don't miss any spots because this acts as a sealant so the bread does not become soggy). On three slices of bread place the cucumber slices, making sure the bread is well covered. Salt and pepper each. Cover with the remaining slices of buttered bread. Trim the crusts. Cut each sandwich into four pieces.

Hint: Make your cuts diagonally from corner to corner, and you'll end up with four triangles.

Alternative: Prepare each sandwich with only one slice of bread and serve these open faced with a tiny sprig of parsley as a garnish.

Nutrient value per serving: 53 calories, 1 g protein, 2 g fat, 9 g carbohydrates, 72 mg sodium, 3 mg cholesterol.

Curried-Egg Sandwiches
12 Servings

8 slices white bread
   unsalted butter
2 eggs, hard-boiled and peeled
⅛ cup mayonnaise, to start
½ teaspoon curry powder

Finely chop the eggs. Stir in mayonnaise and curry powder until all ingredients are well combined and to desired consistency. Spread each slice of bread with a thin coat of butter (don't miss any spots because it acts as a sealer so the bread doesn't get soggy). Divide the egg mixture evenly between four slices of bread and spread evenly. Top each with another slice of bread. With a very sharp serrated knife, trim away all crusts. Cut the sandwiches into three parallel pieces.

Nutrient value per serving: 107 calories, 3 g protein, 6 g fat, 10 g carbohydrates, 133 mg sodium, 40 mg cholesterol.

Lemon Petticoat Tails
20 Servings

Crust:

    1 cup butter
    2 cups all-purpose flour, sifted
    ½ cup powdered sugar, sifted

Filling:

    4 eggs
    2 cups sugar
    ⅓ cup fresh lemon juice
    ¼ cup all-purpose flour
    ½ teaspoon baking powder

Preheat oven to 350°. Grease a 13 x 9-inch baking pan. Cream together the butter and sifted powdered sugar. Blend in flour until thoroughly incorporated. Press dough into baking pan. Bake for 20 to 25 minutes.

While crust is baking, prepare filling. With electric mixer blend together the eggs, sugar, lemon juice, flour, and baking powder. Pour filling over baked crust and bake again uncovered for 20 to 25 minutes. Cool. Dust with powdered sugar. Cut into 20 squares; cut each square diagonally to produce 40 triangular petticoat tails.

Nutrient value per serving: 280 calories, 4 g protein, 10 g fat, 42 g carbohydrates, 116 mg sodium, 67 mg cholesterol.

Pecan Tartlettes
30 Servings

Basic Dough:
½   cup butter
1   3 ounce package cream cheese
1   cup flour
1   tablespoon sugar

Pecan Filling:
2   tablespoons butter, melted
¾   cup brown sugar
1   egg
1½ cups chopped pecans
1   teaspoon vanilla

Preheat oven to 350°.

Crust: Let butter and cream cheese soften to room temperature. Mix together. Add flour and sugar and mix to form a soft dough. Chill at least 1 hour or overnight. Form the dough into 30 walnut-sized balls. Place each ball of dough in each lightly greased mini-muffin cup. Coat your fingers with flour and press them into each dough ball, gently forcing the dough up the sides of the muffin cup until it forms a shell.

Filling: Mix all the ingredients until well blended. Fill each unbaked tart shell. Bake for 15 to 20 minutes. Dust tops with powdered sugar when cool.

Nutrient value per serving: 124 calories, 1 g protein, 10 g fat, 7 g carbohydrates, 66 mg sodium, 24 mg cholesterol.

Scones
8 Servings

Scones are a quick bread similar to biscuits. The recipe originated in Scotland where the name is pronounced "scawn" rather than "scoan." Scones are served throughout Britain, often accompanied by clotted (or Devonshire) cream in addition to butter and jam. There are many varieties of scones, but this is the most basic, classic version.

- 1¼　cups flour
- 1½　teaspoons baking powder
- ¼　cup unsalted butter, cold
- 3　tablespoons sugar
- ⅓　cup whipping cream

Preheat oven to 425°. Combine flour, baking powder, and salt in medium bowl. Cut butter into pieces. Using a pastry blender, two knives, or fingers, work the butter into the dry ingredients until particles are about the size of small peas.

Add sugar. Toss with fork to blend. Add cream, stirring mixture with fork until ingredients begin to hold together. Gather into ball, place on lightly floured surface, and knead gently 10 to 12 times.

Pat dough into a 6-inch circle. Cut into 8 wedges. Place on ungreased baking sheet, slightly apart so sides will crisp. Bake for 12 to 15 minutes until tops are light golden brown.

Remove scones from oven and transfer to kitchen towel placed over a wire rack. Cover scones loosely with remainder of towel and cool 30 minutes before serving.

Currant or raisin scones: Add ½ cup currants or raisins to flour mixture.

Lemon scones: Add 1½ teaspoons grated lemon zest to flour mixture and 1 teaspoon lemon juice to whipping cream.

Nutrient value per serving: 176 calories, 23 g protein, 10 g fat, 20 g carbohydrates, 71 mg sodium, 29 mg cholesterol.

Shortbread
8 Servings

  2 sticks unsalted butter, at room temperature
  ½ cup powdered sugar, sifted
  2 cups all-purpose flour, sifted
  ¼ teaspoon salt

Preheat the oven to 350°. Lightly grease a baking sheet or line it with parchment paper. In a large mixing bowl (or the bowl of an electric mixer) cream the butter until fluffy (at least 2 full minutes). Gradually add the sifted powdered sugar and beat until well combined. Add the flour and salt, mixing only until incorporated, making sure you do not overmix.

On a well-sugared surface, roll out the dough until about ¼ inch thick. Using a small biscuit cutter or sharp knife, cut the dough into rounds, triangles, or other appropriate shapes and transfer them to the baking sheet with a large spatula. Bake for 20 to 25 minutes. The shortbread should be firm but not brown. Remove shortbread while it is still a very pale yellow color. Cool on a rack.

Nutrient value per serving: 167 calories, 3 g protein, 3 g fat, 31 g carbohydrates, 74 mg sodium, 8 mg cholesterol.

The Potluck Revival

Probably nothing in our culture could be considered more down-home, humble, or blasé than the all-American potluck supper, also known as the gathering of the covered-dishes-with-masking-tape-labels.

The spendy 1980s encouraged a far more dignified approach to group dining—The Dinner Party, complete with all of the glitz and expense of fabulous entertaining.

I grew up in the home of a minister, which is my one and only qualification as a potluck aficionado. I know that kids tend to get things mixed up, but I would've sworn "Thou shalt gather regularly for potluck suppers, and the children shalt take only one dessert" was somewhere in the commandments.

In the beginning, the potluck supper represented a surprise at its finest; thus the name pot*luck*. In time, the potluck supper regulations were expanded in an effort to do away with some of the luck. If your last name started with A–H you were to bring a main dish, I–N a salad, and O–Z dessert. Single people could bring rolls, which explained their singleness. They didn't know how to cook. These changes made only a slight improvement because there's just so much you can do to stretch a pound of ground meat and end up with something that travels well.

Potluck dinners always produced a lot of macaroni and cheese, assortments of pasta, meat swimming in variations of greasy liquids, countless forms of gelatin mutations, cakes in pans with sliding lids, and of course, watered-down Kool-Aid. We didn't eat. We took on ballast.

Something remarkable happened early in the 1970s. Someone invented the chicken broccoli casserole. An epidemic broke out across the country as everyone who was sick of spaghetti switched over to the latest in beige and green cuisine. I've nearly forgotten my last potluck, except of course for the eighteen broccoli casseroles and the room temperature instant iced tea. However, resistant as I tend to be in these belt-tightening times, I am more than ready to participate in a potluck revival.

Good Things about Potluck Suppers

- In exchange for bringing one thing you get a full meal.
- It's a good way to unload stuff that's been in the pantry for years because no one in the family really likes it.
- You get to check out others' culinary skills.
- You get to eat things you'd never indulge in at home.
- You get to be with your friends.
- It's a cheap meal out.

Bad Things about Potluck Suppers

- Nothing on your plate is remotely related, and when it all runs together, everything ends up tasting the same.

- People unload stuff that's been in the pantry for years because no one in their family really likes it.
- The warm things are cold, and the cold things are warm.
- Long on function, short on aesthetics.

The Potluck Dinner Party

Combining the benefits of the potluck with the dignity of a dinner party must surely be the frugal wave of the future. Somehow the result should be economical yet elegant.

A more organized and well-planned potluck makes all the difference in the world. The host (you, I presume?) has the freedom to create the menu and the responsibility to make sure exact instructions are communicated to each contributing guest. I suggest that you might start with recipes from this book or pick out an entire menu from a great cookbook that focuses on the art of entertaining. Let me make a suggestion: Rather than assume each of your contributors is a fairly decent cook, assume that they don't know too much. Write out the instructions clearly. Don't skip the smallest step or assume the other person should know how to prepare a basic béchamel. Leave nothing to chance. If you prefer that no substitutions are made and the ingredients remain exactly as printed, be sure to say so.

Rules of Etiquette for the Host

Make up the guest list. The ideal-sized group is eight to twelve because few homes can comfortably accommodate more than twelve dinner guests. Most sets of dishes and flatware come in settings of eight to twelve, and food prepared for this number usually fits easily in one container.

Come up with a theme. The sky is the limit. Think in terms of color, ethnic foods, special occasions, and what you already have in the way of tablecloths, dishes, and stemware. Get ideas from magazines. Each time your mind wanders into territory requiring expenditures, jerk yourself back to reality. Your goal is economical elegance.

Create a menu. Plan every detail from appetizer to dessert. Write down recipes including detailed instructions. Plan portions carefully. Visualize how the entire menu will look when assembled on your table. Are the colors not the same but complementary? Will you have a pleasing array of flavors and a variety of textures? Are the dishes easily served, or will you need additional dishes to accommodate a soup or ragout?

Visualize and plan the presentation. Decide exactly how your buffet or guest table will look. Perhaps you want everything served in clear dishes or on crystal platters. You'll get a lot of laughs if you request all food arrive in and be served in Tupperware. Let your mind wander, and you'll come up with all kinds of clever and unique methods of service. How about fine china? Everyone has some unique piece stashed away in a cupboard just aching to be called into service.

Invite guests. Send or deliver the invitations and assign each invited guest or couple a portion of the meal. Be sure to include the recipe, your preference of serving dish, and the number of guests it should feed. Be clear about whether children are invited.

Assign as much as possible. As the host, you will have plenty to do and provide without being responsible for an appetizer, entrée, salad, or dessert. The whole idea is to keep the cost of entertaining affordable.

Remain flexible. This kind of hosting requires giving up a great deal of control. To imagine that everything will arrive in perfect condition exactly as you might have prepared it yourself is pure folly. Lower your expectations a bit and go with the flow. The world will not come to an end if the entrée arrives scorched. Simply inform the group this is the latest in blackened fare.

Rules of Etiquette for the Guests

Arrive. Once you have committed to attending, nothing short of a note from your undertaker should prevent your appearance.

Arrive on time. You can only imagine the stress you'll cause if you show up an hour late with the appetizers.

Follow instructions to the letter. If you are requested to provide a green salad with red onions, cherry tomatoes, sliced mushrooms, black olives, and croutons in a clear glass salad bowl, don't show up with red Jell-O in swirly-orange Melmac.

Be thorough. Bring everything necessary for your assigned portion of the meal, including the salad dressing, butter, sauce, or garnish. Don't depend on your host to have your finishing touches on hand.

Leave as little as possible to be done on location. Of course some aspects of food preparation must be left until the last moment, i.e. carving meat or tossing salad, but do all you can ahead of time. Don't plan to cook, prepare, or assemble after your arrival.

Do not ask to take your leftovers home. Etiquette dictates that all leftovers stay at the party location. However, if the host offers, feel free to take home what's left of what you brought.

Be a good sport. If you're asked to tint the gravy blue in order to conform with an All Blue Party, just do it. If the host asks that you dress in keeping with the dinner party theme, go ahead; be brave. Anyone can put up with a grass skirt for a few hours.

Offer to reciprocate. If you are a guest, and depending upon the success of the guest mix, you may want to host this same group at a future potluck dinner party.

Since most people appreciate being needed and prefer to help out, the potluck dinner party, or luncheon, or baby shower, or wedding reception (whoops, have I gone too far?) makes far more than just economic sense. It makes people sense.

A Last Resort Dinner

A host is like a general; it takes a mishap to reveal his genius.
—Horace

If it has never happened to you, it will. Just plan on it, be as prepared as possible, and then forget about it.

The scenario: You finally get up your courage to invite the boss and her husband over for dinner. You've planned the perfect menu, designed a killer table setting, envisioned the evening for weeks. The day arrives, you pick up the freshest ingredients, and everything looks great. They will be arriving at 6:00 P.M. It's 4:00 P.M. and everything's on track. And then it happens. Your worst nightmare. You burn the entrée beyond repair, the potatoes have turned to wallpaper paste, the bread dough has completely refused to rise and to top it all off, the sink has backed up and the superintendent is gone for the weekend. They'll be here in exactly twenty-five minutes, and you're sweating bullets.

And then you remember your First Aid Kit—the one you dutifully put together upon reading chapter 2 (look back on page 31). It was a pure stroke of genius that prompted you to tuck each of those ingredients away just in case you ever had a day like today.

The Last Resort meal should take about twenty to twenty-five minutes from the time you discover your regular dinner is ruined until you sit down at the table.

Menu
Seafood on Biscuits
Asparagus
Poached Fruit in Vanilla Sauce with Whipped Topping .

Ingredients
biscuit mix
1 12-ounce can evaporated milk
2 cans shrimp
¼ teaspoon garlic powder or seasoned salt
1 tablespoon sour cream
1 can clam chowder
½ teaspoon pepper
1 can asparagus
1 box instant vanilla pudding mix
1 large can pears or peaches
2 tablespoons favorite flavored syrup
paprika

Optional:
whole milk
flour
canned hollandaise sauce
butter
sugar
fresh vegetables for garnish

First, heat the oven to the temperature given on the biscuit mix box. While the oven is heating, open your can of evaporated milk and put ½ cup of it into a bowl you can whip it in. Put the bowl and your beaters (whether electric or hand) into the freezer for later.

Now, make the biscuit dough following the recipe on the box. If your emergency evaporated milk is the only milk you have, make the biscuits using water. The topping is rich enough that it won't matter all that much. Don't bother to roll out perfect rounds, however; they'll be buried under shrimp. Instead, divide the dough into heaps (two per person) on a floured board. You can use biscuit mix if you're out of flour. Roll each heap into a rough ball and flatten it gently until ½ inch thick. Put them on a greased cookie sheet and into the oven. Bake according to package directions.

While the biscuits are baking, open the two cans of shrimp, dump them into a strainer or colander, and rinse them under cold running water. Set them to drain. Put the clam chowder in a saucepan over low heat. Mix the remaining evaporated milk with an equal amount of water (no need to be exact about this) and measure out the amount you'll need for the vanilla pudding sauce—½ cup less than called for in the pudding directions. Dump the rest of the milk into the chowder and stir. Stir in the shrimp, one tablespoon of sour cream, ½ teaspoon of pepper, and ¼ teaspoon of garlic salt or seasoned salt. Now you have to use your judgment. If the creamed shrimp is too thick, thin it out with a little water (or milk, or cream, if you have it; even sour cream will work just fine).

Now start warming the asparagus. If you wish, you can warm up the hollandaise for the asparagus, but I tend to think that would make too many sauces and too mushy a meal.

Now start making the dessert. Drain the fruit and put it in a saucepan. Mix the instant vanilla pudding using ½ cup less milk than called for in the instructions on the box. Add 2 tablespoons of your favorite flavored syrup, pour it over the fruit and set it over very low heat to warm. By now the biscuits are ready. Split them. Butter them, if you wish, but it's not necessary. Top them with the creamed shrimp. Do you have anything fresh you can garnish this with? Parsley? A wedge of tomato? A few snippets of green onion? No? How about a shake of paprika, then?

Serve with the asparagus.

You'll have to get up in 10 minutes and turn off the fruit. Cover it, and let it just sit there until you're ready for it. When you are, make the topping by whipping the well-chilled evaporated milk. When it's at the soft peak stage, beat in 3 rounded tablespoons of sugar, if you have it. Divide the fruit into serving dishes, spoon on the topping, and serve at once.

Congratulations! You have just survived a total disaster![1]

---

1. "A Last Resort Dinner" excerpted from *How to Repair Food,* copyright © 1987 by Marina and John Bear, by permission of Ten Speed Press, P.O. Box 7123, Berkeley, CA 94707.

$\mathscr{R}$esources

Sales of food by mail have grown to over two billion dollars in the past few years, which certainly indicates there's a real increase in food savvy and demand for authentic ingredients. Each of the following mail order companies offers a catalog.

Mail Order—Food Products

Adagio Teas—gourmet tea from around the world, teapots, and accessories
877-232-4468; www.discovertea.com

Bickford Flavors—flavorings
Cleveland, OH, 216-531-6006; price sheet

Caviarteria Inc.—caviar and gourmet foods
New York, NY, 800-422-8427; catalog

The CMC Company—gourmet seasonings, ethnic foods
Avalon, NJ, 800-262-2780; catalog

Cooking.com—specialty goods, cookware, resources, and website links
800-663-8810; www.cooking.com

Cortland Health Foods—organic and natural foods
Cortland, NY, 607-756-8811; catalog

Jaffe Bros., Inc.—organically grown food
Valley Center, CA, 760-749-1133; catalog

The Maples Fruit Farm, Inc.—dried fruit, nuts, coffee, gift baskets
Chewsville, MD, 301-733-0777; catalog

Northwestern Coffee Mills—coffee, tea, herbs, spices, coffee filters, and coffee flavors
La Pointe, WI, 800-243-5283; catalog

Olde Town Spice Shopper—herbs, spices, and flavorings
St. Charles, MO, 636-916-3600

Palmer's Maple Syrup—maple syrup, cream, and candy
Waitsfield, VT, 802-496-3696; brochure and price list

Pendery's Inc.—herbs, spices, and Mexican seasonings; teas and botanicals
Dallas, TX, 214-741-1870; catalog

Penzey's Spice House—spices, herbs, and seasonings
Waukesha, WI, 800-741-7787; catalog; www.penzeys.com

Rafal Spice Company—coffee, tea, flavorings, cookbooks
Detroit, MI, 313-259-6373; catalog

San Francisco Herb Co.—culinary herbs, teas, spices, and potpourri ingredients
San Francisco, CA, 800-227-4530; catalog

Simpson & Vail, Inc.—coffee, tea, brewing accessories, and gourmet foods
Pleasantville, NY, 800-282-8327; catalog

Spices, Etc.—herbs, spices, tea
Savannah, GA, 800-827-6373; catalog; www.spicesetc.com

The Spice Merchant & Co.—finest coffees, spices, herbs, teas
Jackson Hole, WY, 800-551-5999; catalog; www.orientalcookingsecrets.com

Sultan's Delight, Inc.—Middle Eastern foods and gifts
Brooklyn, NY, 800-852-5046; catalog; www.sultansdelight.com

Upton Tea Imports—world's finest teas
Upton, MA, 800-234-8327; catalog; www.uptontea.com

Wood's Cider Mill—cider jelly and syrups
Springfield, VT, 802-263-5547; catalog; www.woodcidermill.com

Mail Order—Cookware and Equipment

Broadway Panhandler—cookware, cutlery, kitchenware, bakeware
New York, NY, 212-966-3434; price quotes by phone or letter

Chef's Catalog—cookware, cutlery, kitchenware, bakeware
800-338-3232; catalog

Domestications Kitchens and Gardens—kitchen equipment and household items
Hanover, PA, 800-323-6000; catalog; www.domestications-kg.com

Kitchen Etc.—tableware and kitchenware
Exeter, NH, 800-232-4070; catalog; www.kitchenetc.com

Kochtopf—Germany's finest waterless cookware and flatware
Elfters, FL, 800-426-2168; catalog

Professional Cutlery Direct—kitchen cutlery, cookware, cookbooks, kitchen equipment
North Branford, CT, 800-859-6994; catalog; www.cutlery.com

Williams Sonoma—cookware, cookbooks, kitchen equipment, gourmet foods
San Francisco, CA, 800-541-2233; catalog

Zabar's & Co. Inc.—gourmet food, cookware, and housewares
New York, NY, 800-697-6301; catalog; www.zabars.com

Magazines (Available at Newsstands)

Bon Appetit (Condé Nast Publications; monthly)
Provides the gourmet with recipes, and in-depth articles on cuisine-related travel. In addition to preparation instructions aimed at various skill levels, the magazine also features a reader's forum.

Cook's Illustrated (Cook's Illustrated; bi-monthly)
No-nonsense tips for day-to-day cooking; kitchen equipment tests and foot tastings; classic recipes simplified and tested; hand-drawn illustrations with the best "how-to" techniques. Plenty of information about what works, what doesn't, and why.

Fine Cooking (Taunton Press, Inc.; bimonthly)
Written for people who love to cook. Content is strictly devoted to food and food preparation. Material explains the hows and why of a dish, concepts behind recipes, menu ideas, ingredients, and cooking skills and techniques for all levels.

Gourmet (Condé Nast Publications; monthly)
Targeted to the sophisticated epicurean. Features cover culture, history, fine food, as well as art, antiques, travel, and shopping.

Martha Stewart Living (Martha Stewart Living Omnimedia; 10 times/year)
A lifestyle magazine featuring information for people who are actively involved in making their home more beautiful and comfortable, who enjoy entertaining and living well. Each issue includes features on cooking, entertaining, decorating, restoring, remodeling, gardening, traveling, and working.

Sunset Magazine (Sunset Publications Corp.; monthly)
Designed as a functional, how-to magazine for readers interested in Western travel, gardening, building and crafts, and food and entertainment. Emphasis is on the regional coverage of the features in the thirteen Western states.

Cookbooks (Retail Bookstores)

The Best Recipe, Editors of *Cook's Illustrated Magazine,* Boston Common Press, Boston, 1999. This fabulous cookbook contains the 700 best receipes from 7 years of *Cook's Illustrated Magazine.* Each recipe has been tested anywhere from 30 to 80 times to find the very best cooking method. Perfect for both the novice and the expert.

Entertaining, Martha Stewart, Clarkson N. Potter, Inc., New York, 1982. Perhaps her very best work, this book will give you confidence in entertaining. Contains complete menus with recipes, presentation details, etc.

Joy of Cooking, Rombauer and Becker, Bobbs-Merrill Co., New York, 1980. This is an all-round, all-inclusive cookbook that is so foundational none other would be necessary. Desire, perhaps, but not absolutely necessary.

La Technique, Jacques Pépin, Pocket Books, New York, 1976. This is a uniquely illustrated guide to the fundamental techniques of cooking. Excellent!

The Kitchen Survival Guide, Lora Brody, William Morrow and Co., New York, 1992. A hand-holding kitchen primer with 130 recipes to get the beginning cook started.

The Way to Cook, Julia Child, Alfred A. Knopf, New York, 1989. By far, my most favorite cookbook. The book is well illustrated with photos from Julia's viewpoint, not a camerman's. From the most complicated to the most simple, Julia gently teaches and trains.

Miscellaneous (Retail Bookstores)

The Guide to Cooking Schools (Shaw Guides; yearly) Comprehensive resource recommended by leading food publications and organizations. Contains detailed descriptions of more than 1,000 schools, colleges, culinary apprenticeships, cooking vacations, and food organizations worldwide. Programs listed for both career and home cooks.

$\mathcal{R}$ecipe Index

CHAPTER 16—BRITISH CREAM TEA

What Is Cheapskate Monthly?

Cheapskate Monthly is a 12-page newsletter published 12 times a year, dedicated to helping those who are struggling to live within their means find practical and realistic solutions to their financial problems. *Cheapskate Monthly* provides hope, encouragement, inspiration, and motivation to individuals who are committed to financially responsible and debt-free living and provides the highest-quality information and resources possible in a format exclusive of paid advertising. You will find *Cheapskate Monthly* filled with tips, humor, and great information to help you stretch those dollars till they scream!